Fitness Over 60

Workouts For Every Day

2021

N. Rey | darebee.com

Workouts

1. 30-Minute Walk
2. Ankle Recovery
3. Arms & Chest Stretch
4. Arms & Shoulders Stretch
5. Arms & Shoulders
6. Baby Steps
7. Back Fix
8. Back Pain Relief
9. Back To Basics
10. Bad Knees Cardio
11. Below Zero
12. Breathe Easy
13. Breathing
14. Captain On Deck
15. Cardio Grind
16. Cardio Inc
17. Cardio Light
18. Cardio Mill
19. Cardio Sculpt
20. Care Package
21. Catch & Release
22. Centenarian
23. Chest & Lower Back Stretch
24. Couch Potato
25. Cozy Up Sofa
26. Day One
27. Dexterity
28. Easy Does It
29. Energy Boost
30. Everyday Stretching Light
31. Explorer
32. Footwork
33. For Me
34. Fullbody Stretch
35. Glow
36. Hamstring Mobility
37. H & Mobility
38. Healer
39. Health Potion
40. Herald
41. Home
42. Insomnia Yoga
43. Joints Support
44. Kinder
45. Lockdown
46. Lower Back Chair
47. Lower Back
48. Magician
49. Morning Stretch
50. Mr Grumpy
51. Neck & Shoulders
52. No Wrong Answers
53. Once Upon A Time
54. One Angry Bird
55. Party
56. Piece Of Cake
57. Porter
58. Posture Perfect
59. Pressure Points
60. Rainmaker
61. Real
62. Recovery
63. Refresh
64. Regenerator
65. Regen
66. Reset Stretch
67. Rest & Rec
68. Rest & Repair
69. Right Side Bed
70. Rookie
71. Rotator Cuff
72. Roundabout
73. Self Care
74. Shoulder Stretch
75. Sitting Fix
76. Slow Burn
77. Something I Can Do
78. Sore Feet
79. Sore Neck
80. Spine Mobility
81. Stapler
82. Starting Point
83. Steamroller
84. Stiff Neck
85. Stronger Arms
86. Sun Salutation Chair
87. Super Easy
88. Tai Chi
89. Toy Soldier
90. Unwind
91. Upperbody Mobility
92. Upperbody Stretch
93. Upperbody Works
94. Vortex
95. Walker
96. Walk It Off
97. Wizard
98. Wrist Pain
99. Yoga Flow
100. Zen

Introduction

Bodyweight training may look easy, but if you are not used to it, it's very far from that. It is just as intense as running and it is just as challenging so if you struggle with it at the very beginning, it's perfectly ok – you will get better at it once you start doing it regularly. Do it at your own pace and take longer breaks if you need to.

You can start with a single individual workout from the collection and see how you feel. If you are new to bodyweight training always start any workout on Level I (level of difficulty).

You can pick any number of workouts per week, usually between 3 and 5 and rotate them for maximum results.

The Manual

Workout posters are read from left to right and contain the following information: grid with exercises (images), number of reps (repetitions) next to each, number of sets for your fitness level (I, II or III) and rest time.

Difficulty Levels:

Level I: normal
Level II: hard
Level III: advanced

SAMPLE WORKOUT

LEVEL I 3 sets LEVEL II 5 sets LEVEL III 7 sets REST up to 2 minutes

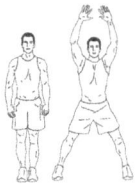 **10** jumping jacks **20** high knees 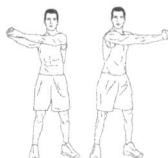 **40** side-to-side chops

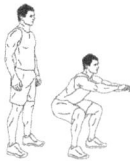 **10** squats 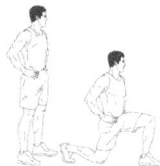 **20** lunges **10-count** plank

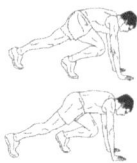 **20** climbers 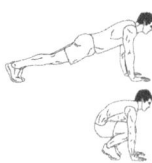 **10** plank jump-ins 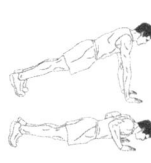 **to failure** push-ups

1 set

10 jumping jacks
20 high knees (10 each leg)
40 side-to-side chops (20 each side)
10 squats
20 lunges (10 each leg)
10-count plank (hold while counting to 10)
20 climbers (10 each leg)
10 plank jump-ins
to failure push-ups (your maximum)

Up to 2 minutes rest between sets
30 seconds, 60 seconds or 2 minutes - it's up to you.

"Reps" stands for repetitions, how many times an exercise is performed. Reps are usually located next to each exercise's name. Number of reps is always a total number for both legs / arms / sides. It's easier to count this way: e.g. if it says 20 climbers, it means that both legs are already counted in - it is 10 reps each leg.

Reps to failure means to muscle failure = your personal maximum, you repeat the move until you can't. It can be anything from one rep to twenty, normally applies to more challenging exercises. The goal is to do as many as you possibly can.

The transition from exercise to exercise is an important part of each circuit (set) - it is often what makes a particular workout more effective. Transitions are carefully worked out to hyperload specific muscle groups more for better results. For example if you see a plank followed by push-ups it means that you start performing push-ups right after you finished with the plank avoiding dropping your body on the floor in between.

There is no rest between exercises - only after sets, unless specified otherwise. You have to complete the entire set going from one exercise to the next as fast as you can before you can rest.

What does "up to 2 minutes rest" mean: it means you can rest for up to 2 minutes but the sooner you can go again the better. Eventually your recovery time will improve naturally, you won't need all two minutes to recover - and that will also be an indication of your improving fitness.

Recommended rest time:

Level I: 2 minutes or less
Level II: 60 seconds or less
Level III: 30 seconds or less

Video Exercise Library
http://darebee.com/video

The workouts are organized in alphabetical order so you can find the workouts you favor easier and faster.

warmup

by DAREBEE © darebee.com

Repeat each exercise for 10-20 seconds then move on to the next one.

1 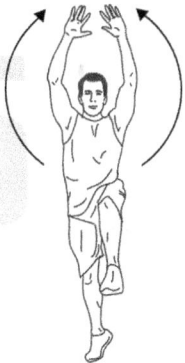 2 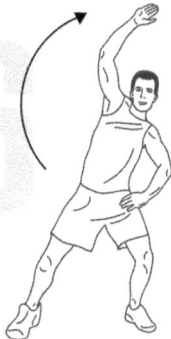 3 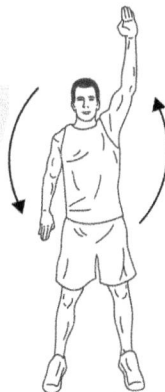 4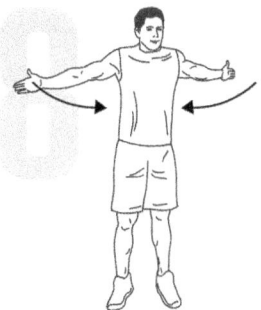

5 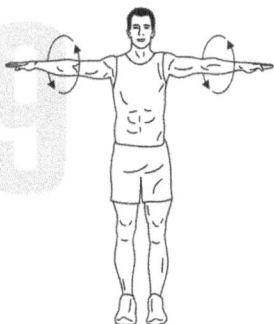 6 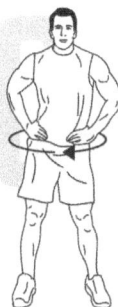 7 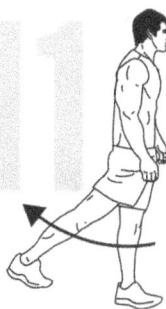 8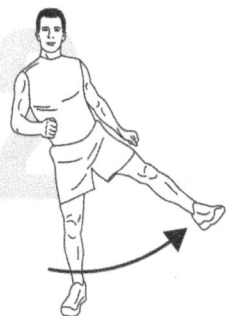

9 10 11 12

#1

30-Minute Walk Workout

Focus: Cardiovascular system

Benefits: body fat reduction, endurance

30-MINUTE
WALK

WORKOUT by DAREBEE © darebee.com

Repeat 5 times in total

60sec march steps

15sec step jacks

60sec march steps

15sec step jacks

60sec march steps

15sec step jacks

60sec march steps

15sec step jacks

60sec rest

#2

Ankle Recovery Workout

Focus: Ankle strength and agility

Benefits: recovery and rehabilitation, pain relief, mobility

ankle
recovery

DAREBEE WORKOUT © darebee.com

30 seconds each exercise.

up and down tilts

side-to-side tilts

toe curls

calf stretch

single leg balance

elevated calf raises

#3

Arms & Chest Stretch Workout

Focus: Upper body range of motion

Benefits: tension relief, muscle soreness reduction

arms & chest stretch

by DAREBEE
© darebee.com
20 seconds each exercise.

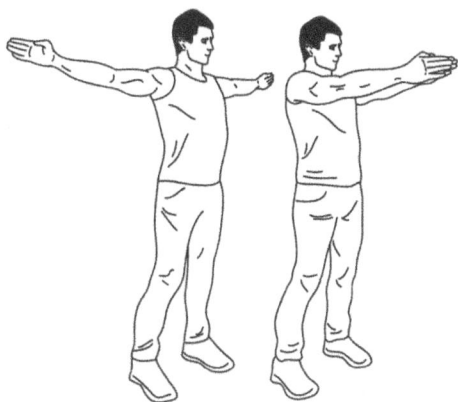

chest expansions

side-to-side torso twists

overhead stretch

chest expansions

side-to-side tilts

tricep stretches

#4

Arms & Shoulders Stretch Workout

Focus: Upper body

Benefits: tension relief, muscle soreness reduction

arms & shoulder stretch

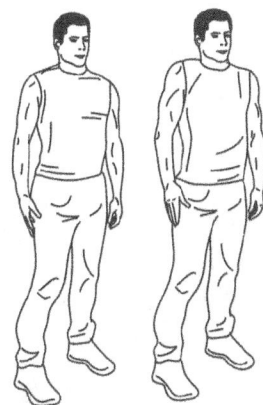

by DAREBEE
© darebee.com
20 seconds each exercise.

bicep extensions

bicep extensions
both arms

elbow clicks

tricep expansions

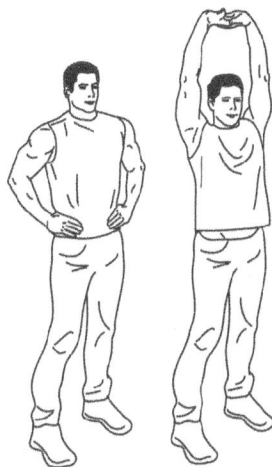

shoulder stretch

shoulder rotations

#5

Arms & Shoulders Workout

Focus: Upper body strength and dexterity

Benefits: tendon strength, tone and streamline

ARMS & SHOULDERS

DAREBEE WORKOUT © darebee.com

LEVEL I 3 sets **LEVEL II** 5 sets **LEVEL III** 7 sets **REST** up to 2 minutes

10 bicep extensions

10 side shoulder taps

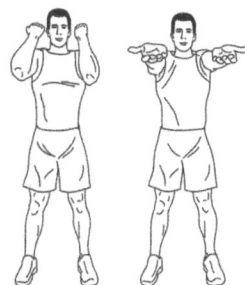

10 bicep extensions

10 arm circles

10 bicep extensions

10 arm circles

10 bicep extensions

10 side shoulder taps

10 bicep extensions

#6

Baby Steps Workout

Focus: Cardiovascular system

Benefits: body fat reduction, endurance

BABY STEPS

DAREBEE WORKOUT
© darebee.com

LEVEL I 3 sets
LEVEL II 5 sets
LEVEL III 7 sets
REST up to 2 minutes

10 march steps

10 scissor chops

10 arm scissors

10 march steps

10 chest expansions

10 arm circles

#7

Back Fix Workout

Focus: Lower back

Benefits: tension relief, pain reduction and pain management

back fix

DAREBEE WORKOUT © darebee.com
Hold each pose for 20 seconds.

shoulder shrug

shoulder stretch

side bend

sea horse

seated twist

wide leg fold

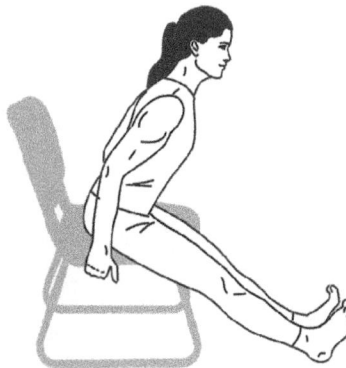

hamstring stretch

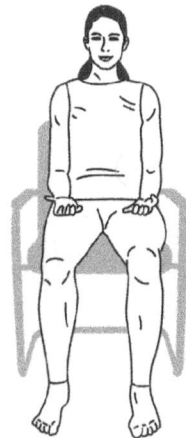

fall back

#8

Back Pain Relief Workout

Focus: Lower and upper back

Benefits: tension relief, muscle soreness reduction, agility

stretching for
back pain
relief

by DAREBEE © darebee.com

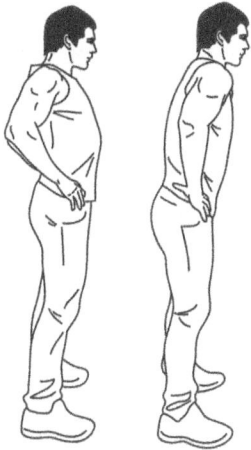

10 back and forth arches

10 alternate shoulder raises

10 shoulder rotations

10 torso twists

10 side-to-side bends

10 torso rotations

#9

Back To Basics Workout

Focus: Cardiovascular system

Benefits: body fat reduction, endurance

Back to Basics

DAREBEE WORKOUT © darebee.com

LEVEL I 3 sets **LEVEL II** 5 sets **LEVEL III** 7 sets **REST** up to 2 minutes

20 step jacks

20 raised arm circles

20 step jacks

20 chest expansions

20 step jacks

20 alt chest expansions

#10

Bad Knees Cardio Workout

Focus: Cardiovascular system and fascia

Benefits: body fat reduction at low impact, agility

BAD KNEES CARDIO

DAREBEE WORKOUT © darebee.com

LEVEL I 3 sets **LEVEL II** 5 sets **LEVEL III** 7 sets **REST** up to 2 minutes

20 step jacks

10 side jacks

20 step jacks

20 march steps

10 side leg raises

20 march steps

#11

Below Zero Workout

Focus: Core stability

Benefits: body fat reduction, tendon strength and mobility

Below Zero

DAREBEE WORKOUT © darebee.com

LEVEL I 3 sets **LEVEL II** 5 sets **LEVEL III** 7 sets **REST** up to 2 minutes

4 sit to stand

Hold on for support if needed
10 side leg raises

Hold on for support if needed
10 back leg raises

10 step jacks

4 side bends

4 hip rotations

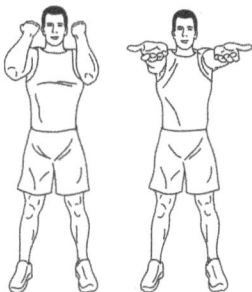

10 bicep extensions

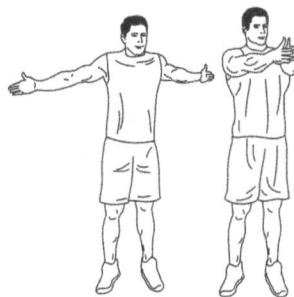

10 chest expansions

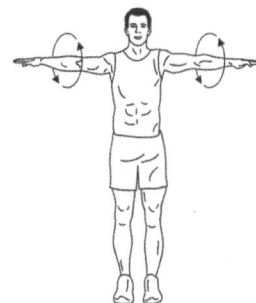

10 arm circles

#12

Breathe Easy Workout

Focus: Upper body mobility

Benefits: lung health, metabolic health, range of motion

breathe
easy

WORKOUT by © darebee.com

Arms above your head

1) Breathe in deep;
2) Hold to count of five;
3) Exhale to count of five.

Repeat 5 times in total.

Arm Raises

1) Breathe in
as you raise your arms;
2) Exhale on the way down.

Repeat 5 times in total.

Calf Raises

1) Breathe in as you rise;
2) Hold to count of five;
3) Exhale as you drop down.

Repeat 5 times in total.

Shoulder Stretches
arms behind your back

1) Breathe in as you stretch;
2) Hold to count of five;
3) Exhale as you relax.

Repeat 5 times in total.

#13

Breathing Workout

Focus: Lung health

Benefits: lung health, concentration, metabolic health

Breathing Workout

by DAREBEE © darebee.com

Breathe in slowly, hold to a slow count of ten then exhale slowly. Repeat 3 times.

Take ten rapid breaths. Hold without breathing to the count of twenty.

Breathe in and lean back, breathe out and lean forward. Repeat 3 times.

Breathe in fast, breathe out fast. Hold for count of three. Repeat 3 times.

#14

Captain On Deck Workout

Focus: Upper body dexterity

Benefits: strength and tone, range of motion

CAPTAIN ON DECK

DAREBEE WORKOUT © darebee.com

LEVEL I 3 sets **LEVEL II** 5 sets **LEVEL III** 7 sets **REST** up to 2 minutes

10 arm raises

10 arm extensions

10 arm scissors

10 shoulder taps

10 bicep extensions

10 side shoulder taps

#15

Cardio Grind Workout

Focus: Cardiovascular system

Benefits: body fat reduction, endurance, hip tendon strength

Cardio Grind

DAREBEE WORKOUT © darebee.com

repeat 3 times with 2 minutes rest in between

20 march steps

10 elbow clicks

10 step elbow clicks

20 march steps

10 shoulder taps

10 step shoulder taps

20 march steps

10 bicep extensions

10 step bicep extensions

#16

Cardio Inc Workout

Focus: Agility

Benefits: improved range of motion

Cardio Inc.

DAREBEE WORKOUT © darebee.com
repeat 3 times with 2 minutes rest in between

20 step jacks

4 step side jacks

4 chest expansions

20 step jacks

4 step side jacks

4 chest expansions

20 step jacks

4 step side jacks

4 chest expansions

#17

Cardio Light Workout

Focus: Cardiovascular system

Benefits: body fat reduction, endurance, improved lower body strength, agility,

cardio light

DAREBEE WORKOUT © darebee.com

LEVEL I 3 sets **LEVEL II** 5 sets **LEVEL III** 7 sets **REST** up to 2 minutes

10 march steps

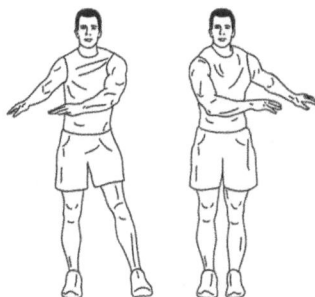

10 step jacks

10 march steps

10 side jacks

10 march steps

10 scissor steps

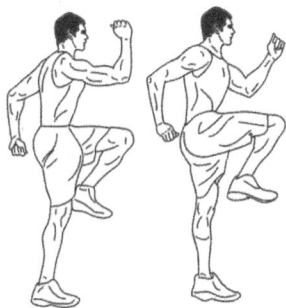

10 march steps

10 side-to-side steps

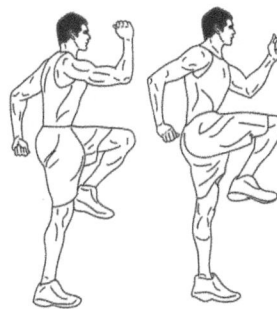

10 march steps

#18

Cardio Mill Workout

Focus: Cardiovascular system

Benefits: endurance, dexterity, balance, posture

Cardio Mill

DAREBEE WORKOUT © darebee.com

repeat 3 times with 2 minutes rest in between

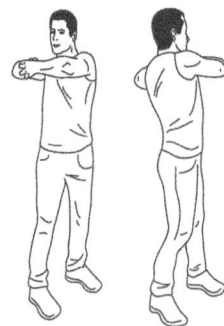

20 side step jacks   **20** alt chest expansions   **4** clasped arm rotations

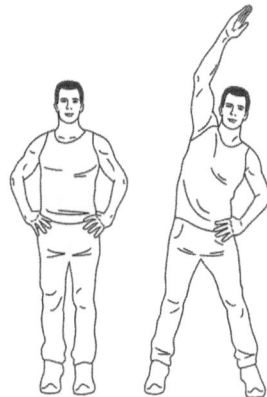

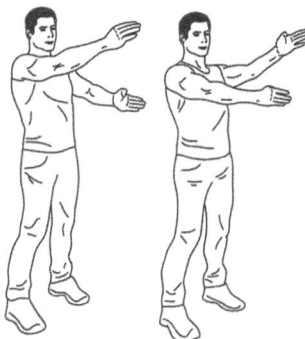

20 side step jacks   **20** chest expansions   **4** clasped arm rotations

20 side step jacks   **20** arm chops   **4** clasped arm rotations

#19

Cardio Sculpt Workout

Focus: Cardiovascular system

Benefits: balance, lower body strength, coordination, agility

Cardio Sculpt

DAREBEE WORKOUT © darebee.com

repeat 3 times with 2 minutes rest in between

20 march steps

10 double punch step

20 march steps

10 twists

20 march steps

10 knee-to-elbows

#20

Care Package Workout

Focus: Stretching

Benefits: flexibility, muscle tension reduction, lower back and pelvic region health

CARE PACKAGE

DAREBEE WORKOUT © darebee.com

10 seconds each stretch

#1 #2 #3 #4 #5

#6 #7 #8 #9 #10

#11 #12 #13 #14

#21

Catch & Release Workout

Focus: Tendon strength

Benefits: flexibility, range of motion, neck stability

Catch & Release

DAREBEE WORKOUT
© darebee.com

overhead clench
20

overhead punches
20

extended clench
20

punches
20

side extended clench
20

torso twists
20

#22

Centenarian Workout

Focus: Agility

Benefits: tendon strength, balance, coordination, posture

THE CENTENARIAN

DAREBEE WORKOUT © darebee.com

LEVEL I 3 sets **LEVEL II** 5 sets **LEVEL III** 7 sets **REST** up to 2 minutes

20 straight back leg swings   **10** hip rotations   **20** alternating chest expansions

20 march jacks   **20** side jacks

#23

Chest & Lower Back Stretch Workout

Focus: Agility

Benefits: lower back health, spine health, flexibility, agility

chest & *lowerback* stretch

by DAREBEE
© darebee.com
20 seconds each exercise.

side bends

forward bends

torso twists

side leg raises

alt chest expansions

chest expansions

#24

Couch Potato Workout

Focus: Range of motion

Benefits: improved posture, agility

couch potato

DAREBEE WORKOUT © darebee.com

20sec overhead clench / unclench

40sec overhead hold

20sec to the side clench / unclench

40sec to the side hold

20sec to the front clench / unclench

40sec to the front hold

#25

Cozy Up Sofa Workout

Focus: Upper body agility

Benefits: improved range of movement, upper body flexibility

cozy up

DAREBEE SOFA WORKOUT ©darebee.com

Hold each stretch and **count to 10**, change sides and hold it again
every time you cozy up on the sofa to stretch your muscles.
and help blood circulation.

1

2

3

4

5

6

#26

Day One Workout

Focus: Cardiovascular system, aerobic capacity

Benefits: increased lower body strength, stronger core and abs

DAY ONE

DAREBEE
WORKOUT
© darebee.com

Level I 3 sets
Level II 5 sets
Level III 7 sets
2 minutes rest

10 forward lunges   **20** bicep extensions   **20** shoulder taps

10 bridges   **10** heel taps   **10** flutter kicks

#27

Dexterity Workout

Focus: Range of motion

Benefits: increased dexterity and upper body control, tendon strength

DEX TERI TY

DAREBEE
WORKOUT
© darebee.com
LEVEL I 3 sets
LEVEL II 4 sets
LEVEL III 5 sets
REST up to 2 minutes

10 arm scissors

10 scissor chops

10 shoulder rotations

10 bicep extensions

10 shoulder taps

30 clench / unclench

#28

Easy Does It Workout

Focus: Tendon strength

Benefits: greater hip flexibility, better posture, stronger neck & lower back

EASY
DOES IT

DAREBEE WORKOUT © darebee.com

LEVEL I 3 sets **LEVEL II** 5 sets **LEVEL III** 7 sets **REST** up to 2 minutes

10 step jacks

20 side leg raises

10 step jacks

20 raised arm circles

10 step jacks

20 raised arm circles

#29

Energy Boost Workout

Focus: Upper body & tendons

Benefits: greater coordination, better balance, improved agility

ENERGY BOOST

DAREBEE WORKOUT © darebee.com

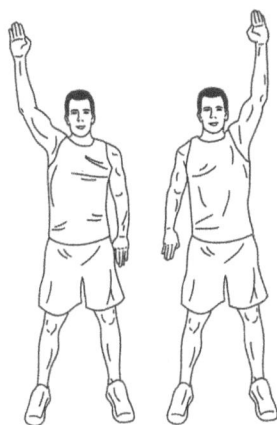

10 alt chest expansions

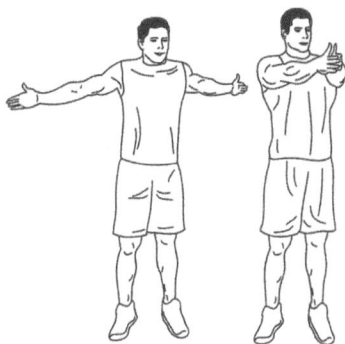

10 chest expansions

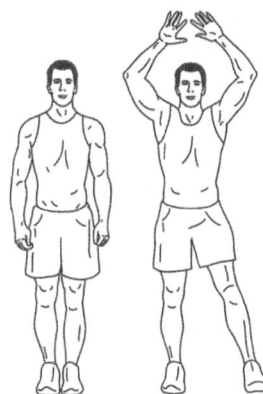

10 step jacks

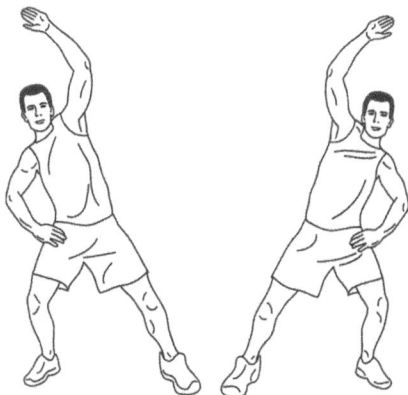

10 side jacks

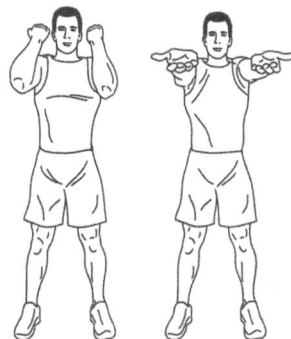

10 bicep extensions

#30

Everyday Stretching Light Workout

Focus: Neck & lower back

Benefits: improved agility, improved posture, better balance

LIGHT EVERYDAY STRETCHING

DAREBEE WORKOUT © darebee.com

Repeat (exercises with arrows) or hold (no arrows) each stretch
30 seconds each - 30 seconds per side

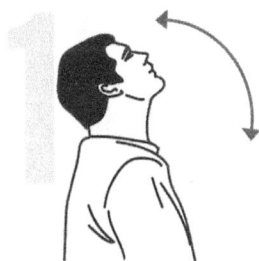

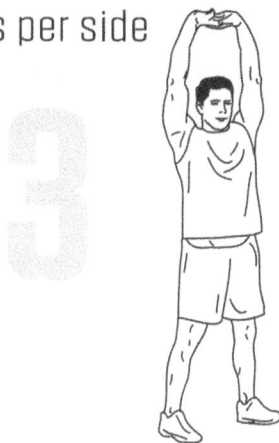

#31

Explorer Workout

Focus: Cardiovascular system & tendons

Benefits: agility, improved posture, resistance to fatigue

EXPLORER

DAREBEE WORKOUT © darebee.com

LEVEL I 3 sets **LEVEL II** 5 sets **LEVEL III** 7 sets **REST** up to 2 minutes

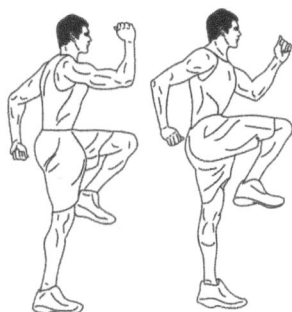

20 march steps

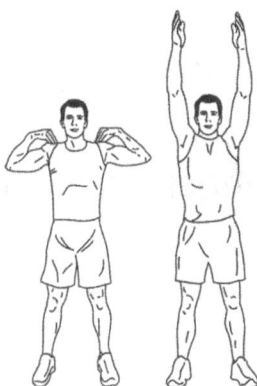

10 shoulder taps

10 bicep extensions

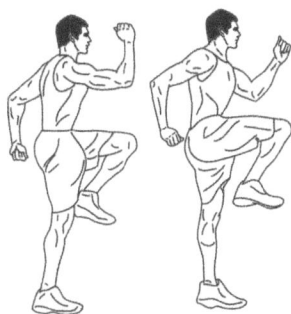

20 march steps

10 scissor chops

10 arm scissors

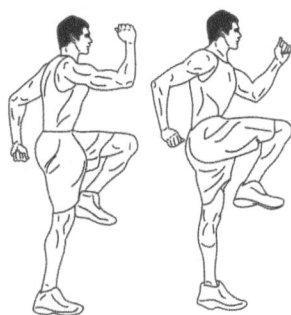

20 march steps

10 chest expansions

10 raised arm circles

#32

Footwork Workout

Focus: Joint health

Benefits: stronger ankles, healthier feet

f👣twork

DAREBEE 2-MINUTE WORKOUT © darebee.com
FOOT SORENESS & TENSION RELIEF;
IMPROVED CIRCULATION & POSTURE
- 20 seconds each -

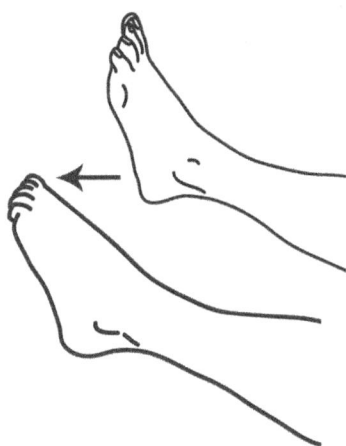

1. forward bends

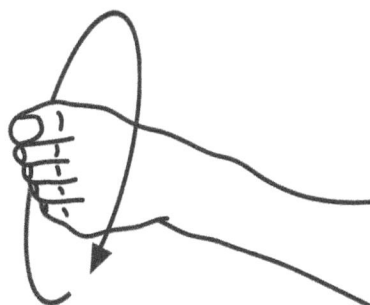

2. rotations

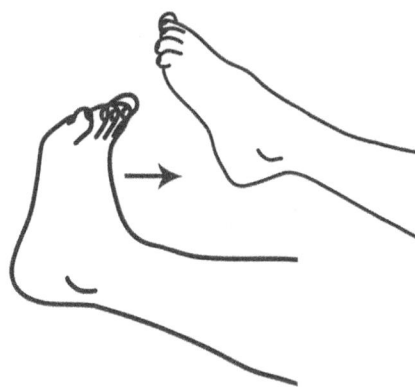

3. forward & backward bends

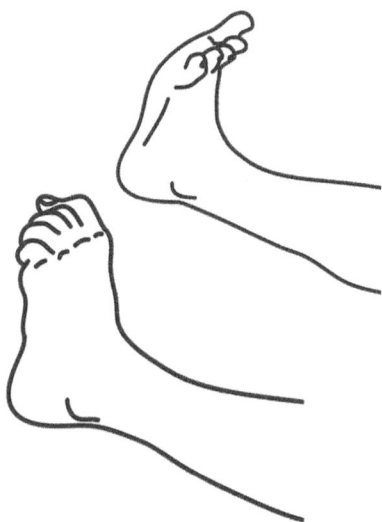

4. clench & unclench

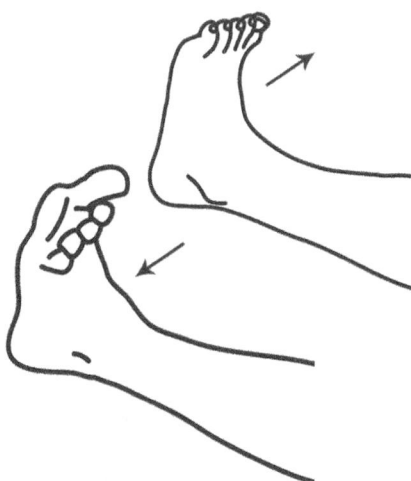

5. side-to-side

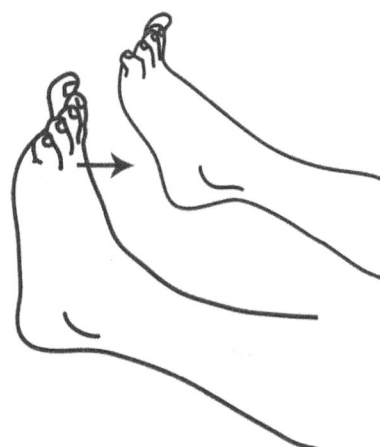

6. toes back bends

#33

For Me Workout

Focus: Lower body

Benefits: stronger legs, improved posture

This one is for me

DAREBEE WORKOUT © darebee.com
5 sets   2 minutes rest between sets

10 knee-to-elbows   **10** side jacks   **6** high squats

6 deadlift & twists   **6** reverse lunges

#34

Fullbody Stretch Workout

Focus: Flexibility

Benefits: improved agility & range of motion

full body stretch

by DAREBEE
© darebee.com

40 seconds each exercise.

neck stretch

shoulder stretch

tricep stretch

pelvic stretch

quad stretch

forward bend

#35

Glow Workout

Focus: Spine health
Benefits: improved agility & posture

GLOW

DAREBEE WORKOUT © darebee.com

Hold each pose for 30 seconds then move on to the next one.
Repeat the sequence again on the other side.

#36

Hamstring Mobility Workout

Focus: Flexibility

Benefits: improved range of motion & knee stability

hamstring
mobility

DAREBEE WORKOUT © darebee.com

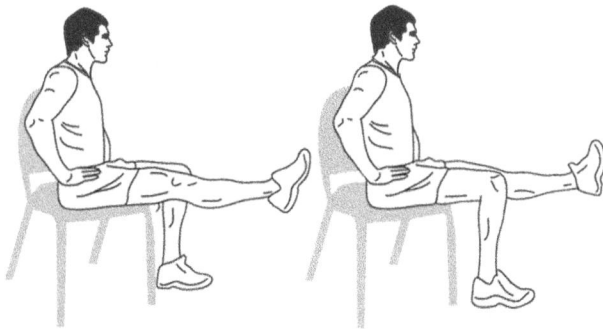

10 leg raises
4 sets in total
30 sec rest in between

10 leg swings
4 sets in total
30 sec rest in between

10 back leg raises
4 sets in total
30 sec rest in between

10-count hamstring stretch
2 sets in total
30 sec rest in between

10-count forward bend
2 sets in total
30 sec rest in between

#37

Hand Mobility Workout

Focus: Wrist joint

Benefits: stronger wrists and hands

hand mobility

DAREBEE WORKOUT © darebee.com
20 seconds each exercise.
Repeat every couple of hours.

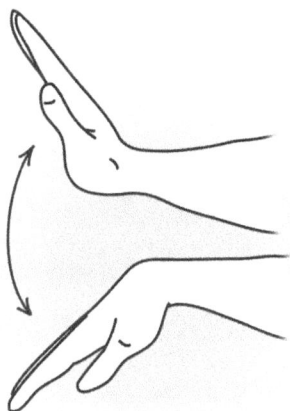

up & down stretch   **up & down side stretch**   **rotations**

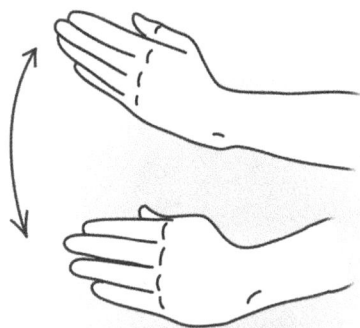

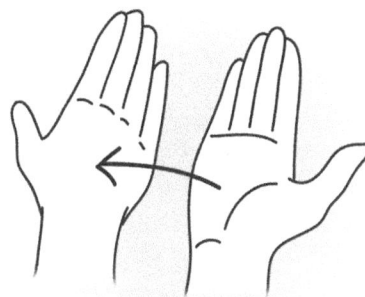

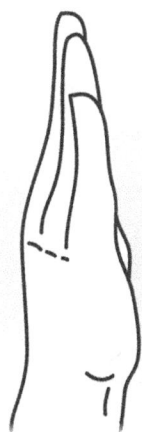

arrow - into - **table top** - into - **straight fist** - into - **claw** - into - **fist**

#38

Healer Workout

Focus: Cardiovascular fitness

Benefits: lower body strength, agility

HEALER

DAREBEE WORKOUT © darebee.com

LEVEL I 3 sets **LEVEL II** 5 sets **LEVEL III** 7 sets **REST** up to 2 minutes

5 calf raises

10 reverse lunges

5 calf raises

10 knee-to-elbows

5 high squats

10 knee-to-elbows

10 arm scissors

10 raised arm circles

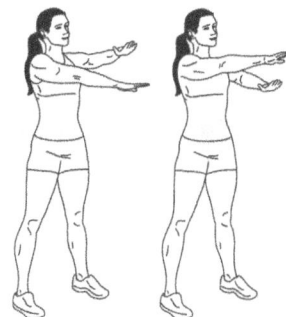

10 arm scissors

#39

Health Potion Workout

Focus: Agility & tendon strength

Benefits: suppleness, posture, endurance

HEALTH POTION
— FULL STRENGTH —

DAREBEE
WORKOUT
© darebee.com
Level I 3 sets
Level II 5 sets
Level III 7 sets
2 minutes rest

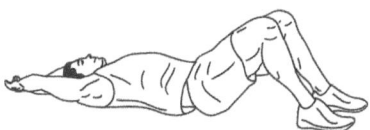

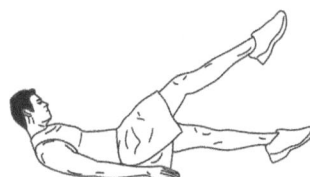

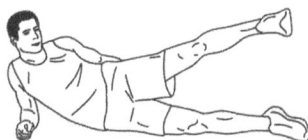

10 bridges

20 side leg raises

10 flutter kicks

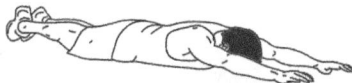

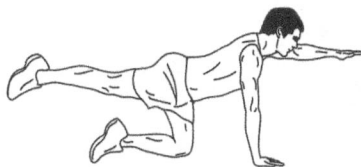

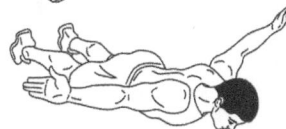

20 alt arm / leg raises

10 superman extensions

10 prone reverse flyes

#40

Herald Workout

Focus: Upper Body

Benefits: improved upper body control

HERALD

DAREBEE WORKOUT © darebee.com

LEVEL I 3 sets **LEVEL II** 5 sets **LEVEL III** 7 sets **REST** up to 2 minutes

10 shoulder taps

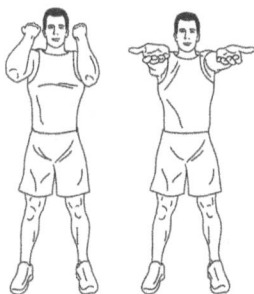

10 bicep extensions

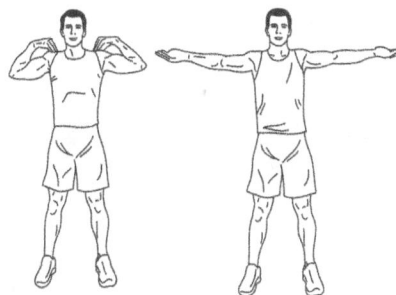

10 arm circles

10 shoulder taps

10 bicep extensions

10 elbow clicks

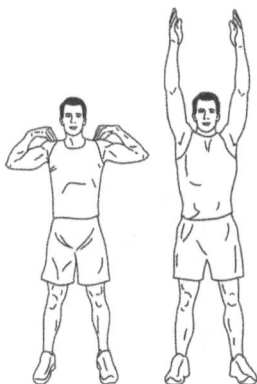

10 shoulder taps

10 bicep extensions

10 side shoulder taps

#41

Home Workout

Focus: Agility

Benefits: stronger lower back, abs, glutes & hips

HOME
WORKOUT

MADE by DAREBEE © darebee.com

Repeat 5 times in total - Rest up to 2 minutes in between

10 hip rotations   **10** step jacks   **10** chest expansions

10 calf raises   **10** march steps

#42

Insomnia Yoga Workout

Focus: agility, flexibility

Benefits: improved circulation, calmness

INSOMNIA
YOGA

DAREBEE WORKOUT © **darebee.com**

Hold each pose for 30 seconds then move on to the next one.

1

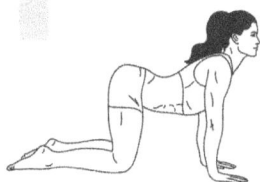

2

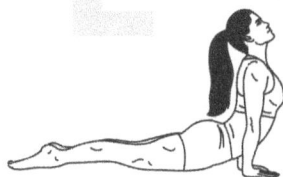

3

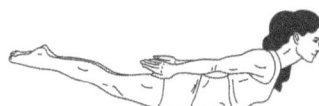

4

5

6

7

8

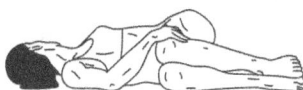

9

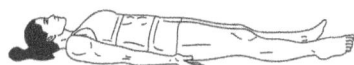

#43

Joints Support Workout

Focus: joint health

Benefits: supple joints

JOINTS
SUPPORT

DAREBEE WORKOUT © darebee.com

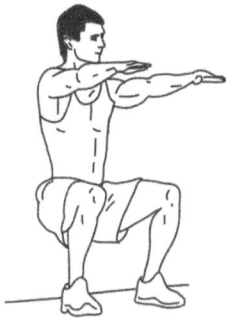

30sec wall sit

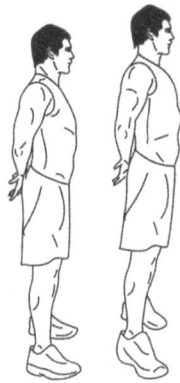

10 calf raises

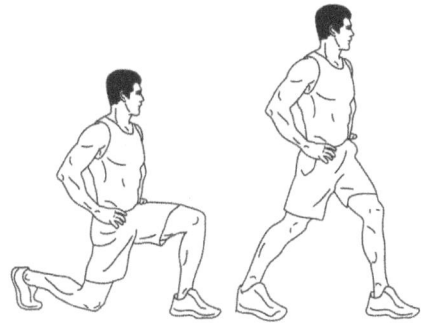

10 split lunges

30sec wall push-up hold

30 raised arm circles

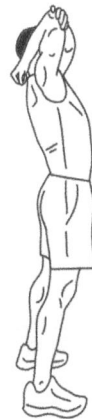

30sec shoulder stretch

#44

Kinder Workout

Focus: cardiovascular health

Benefits: greater body control

KINDER

DAREBEE WORKOUT © darebee.com

LEVEL I 3 sets **LEVEL II** 5 sets **LEVEL III** 7 sets **REST** up to 2 minutes

10 march steps

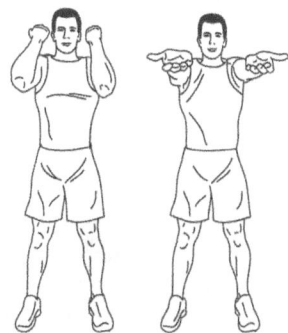

10 raised arm circles

10 march steps

10 arm extensions

10 march steps

10 bicep extensions

#45

Lockdown Workout

Focus: agility, mobility

Benefits: tendon strength

LOCKDOWN

WORKOUT
BY DAREBEE
© darebee.com

Repeat 5 times in total.
Up to 2 minutes rest
between sets.

10 knee-to-elbows

10 step jacks

10 reverse lunges

20 shoulder taps

20 side shoulder taps

20 raised arm circles

#46

Lower Back Chair Workout

Focus: lower back health

Benefits: spine mobility, flexibility

lower **back**

DAREBEE WORKOUT © darebee.com
20 seconds each exercise.

chair edition

knee in stretch

side stretch

knee fold forward stretch

knee-to-elbow stretch

side twist

#47

Lower Back Workout

Focus: agility, spine health

Benefits: flexibility, suppleness

LOWER
BACK

REHAB WORKOUT
© darebee.com
3 sets | 2 minutes rest

5 bottom to heels stretch

10 opposite arm / leg raises

5 back extensions

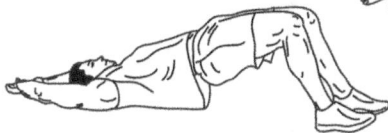

10 bridges

10 knee rolls

#48

Magician Workout

Focus: upper body dexterity

Benefits: improved upper body muscle tone

MAGICIAN

DAREBEE WORKOUT © darebee.com

LEVEL I 3 sets **LEVEL II** 4 sets **LEVEL III** 5 sets **REST** up to 2 minutes

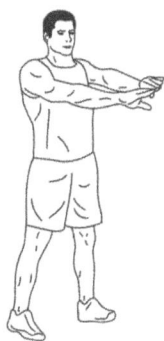

20sec hold

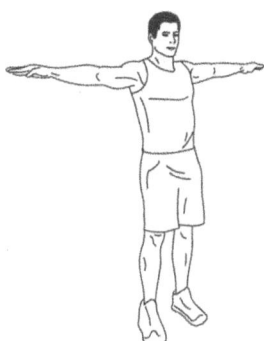

20sec hold

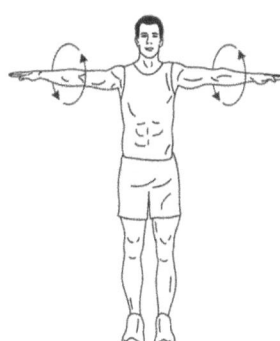

20sec raised arm circles

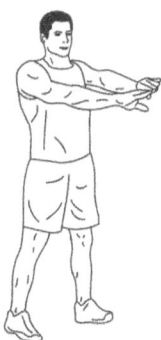

20sec hold

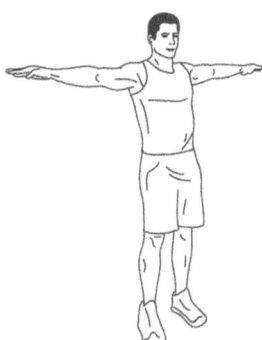

20sec hold

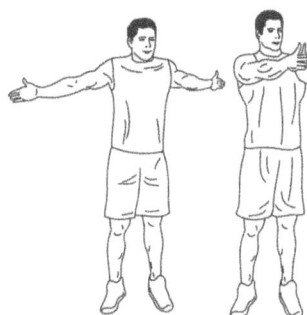

20sec chest expansions

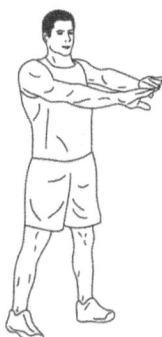

20sec hold

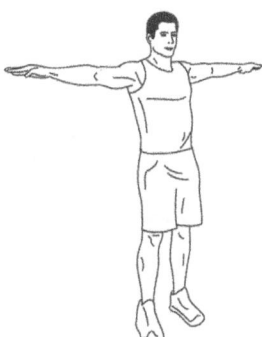

20sec hold

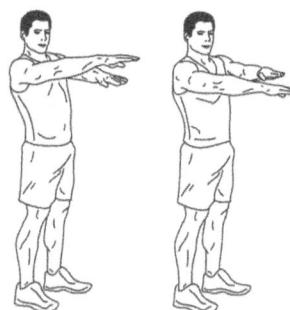

20sec arm scissors

#49

Morning Stretch Workout

Focus: Agility

Benefits: improved range of motion and joint stability

morning
stretch

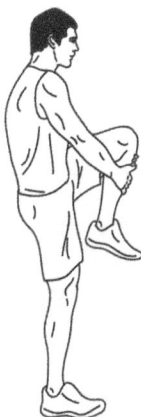

by DAREBEE
© darebee.com
30 seconds each

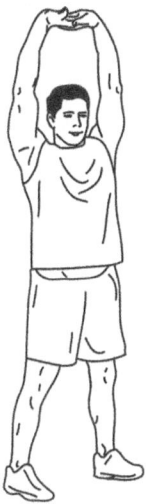

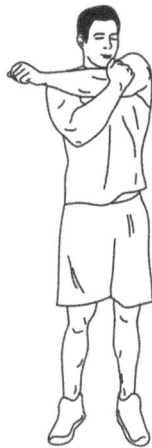

shoulder stretch #1   shoulder stretch #2   upper back stretch   core stretch

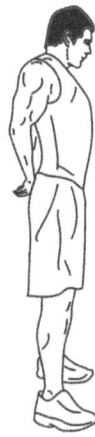

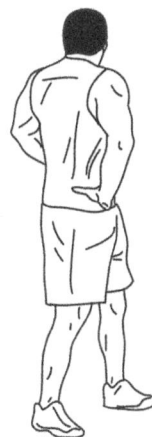

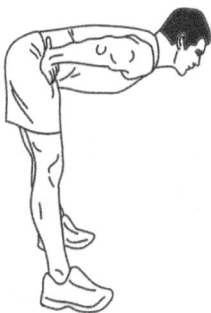

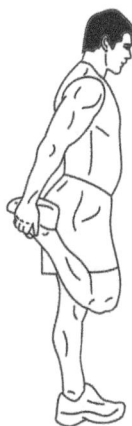

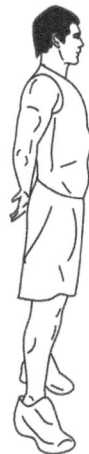

hamstring stretch   glute stretch   quad stretch   calf raise hold

#50

Mr Grumpy Workout

Focus: Mobility

Benefits: improved posture and resistance to fatigue

Mr Grumpy

DAREBEE WORKOUT © darebee.com

LEVEL I 3 sets **LEVEL II** 5 sets **LEVEL III** 7 sets **REST** up to 2 minutes

20 march steps

20 chest expansions

20 march steps

20 bicep extensions

20 march steps

20 shoulder taps

#51

Neck & Shoulders Workout

Focus: Upper body agility

Benefits: improved circulation and range of movement

neck & shoulders

DAREBEE WORKOUT © darebee.com
20 seconds each exercise.

shoulder rotations

side shoulder stretch

cross shoulder stretch

tricep stretch

overhead shoulder stretch

up and down neck stretch

#52

No Wrong Answers Workout

Focus: Shoulders and chest

Benefits: stronger shoulders and pectoral muscles

NO WRONG ANSWERS

DAREBEE WORKOUT © darebee.com

LEVEL I 3 sets **LEVEL II** 5 sets **LEVEL III** 7 sets **REST** up to 2 minutes

10 bicep extensions

10 side shoulder taps

10 shoulder taps

10 scissor chops

10 arm scissors

10 arm circles

#53

Once Upon A Time Workout

Focus: cardiovascular system

Benefits: Stronger muscles, improved coordination

ONCE UPON A TIME

DAREBEE WORKOUT
© darebee.com
LEVEL I 3 sets
LEVEL II 5 sets
LEVEL III 7 sets
REST up to 2 minutes

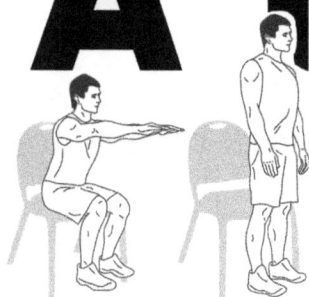

4 sit to stand

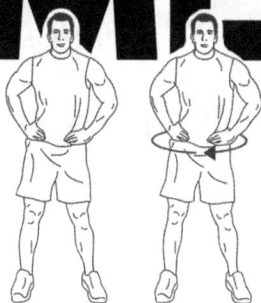

10 hip rotations

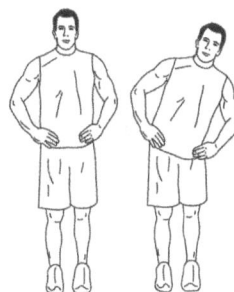

10 side bends

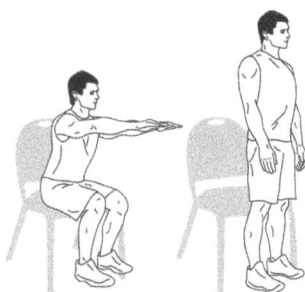

4 sit to stand

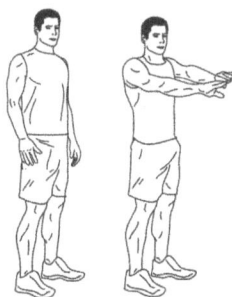

10 arm raises

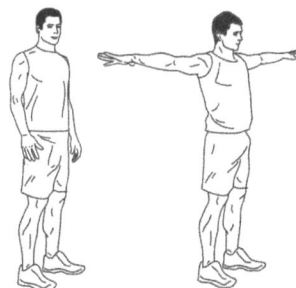

10 side arm raises

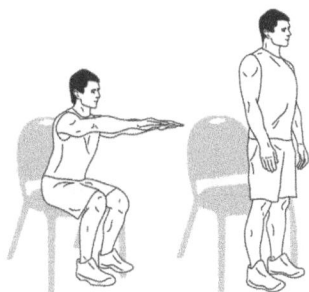

4 sit to stand

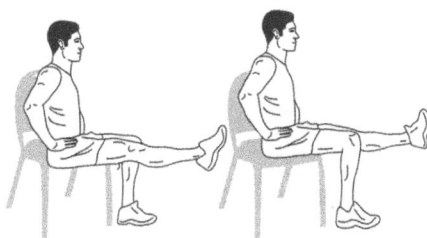

10 leg raises

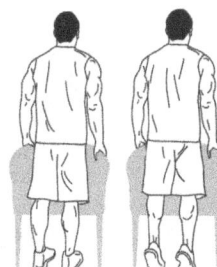

10 calf raises

#54

One Angry Bird Workout

Focus: upper body

Benefits: improved upper body tendon strength & muscle tone

ONE ANGRY BiRD

DAREBEE WORKOUT © darebee.com

LEVEL I 3 sets **LEVEL II** 5 sets **LEVEL III** 7 sets **REST** up to 2 minutes

10 arm circles

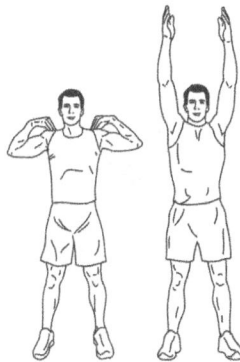

10 scissor chops

10 arm scissors

10 arm circles

10 arm raises

10 chest expansions

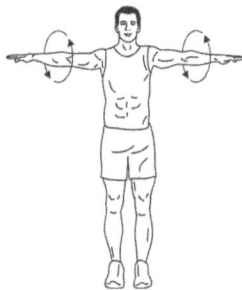

10 arm circles

10 shoulder taps

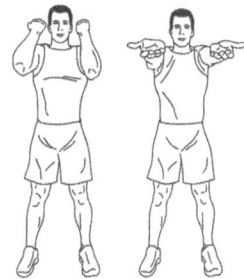

10 bicep extensions

#55

Party Workout

Focus: Agility, mobility

Benefits: improved posture & overall strength

IT'S PARTY TIME

DAREBEE
WORKOUT
© darebee.com

LEVEL I 3 sets
LEVEL II 5 sets
LEVEL III 7 sets
REST up to 2 minutes

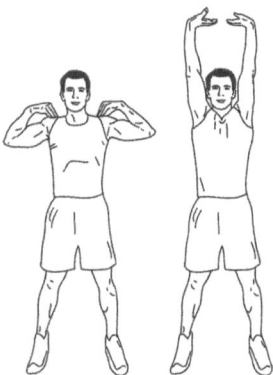

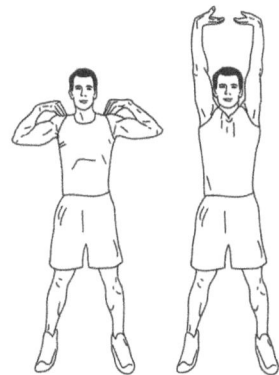

20 shoulder taps

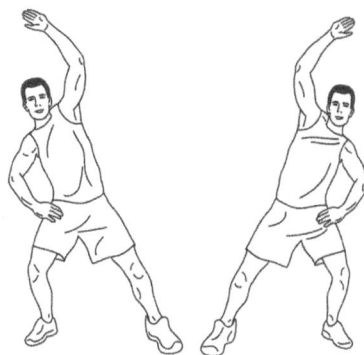

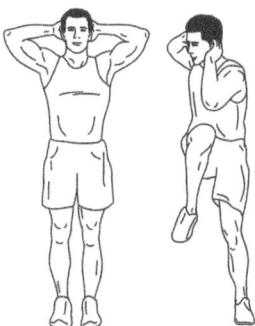

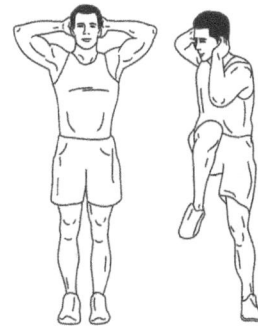

10 side jacks

20 shoulder taps

10 knee-to-elbows

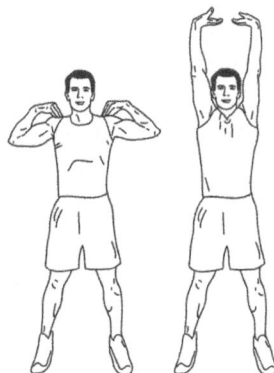

20 shoulder taps

10 knee-to-elbows

#56

Piece Of Cake Workout

Focus: Abs, hips & lower back

Benefits: stronger abs, improved hip strength

PIECE OF CAKE

DAREBEE
WORKOUT
© darebee.com

Level I   3 sets
Level II   4 sets
Level III 5 sets
2 minutes rest

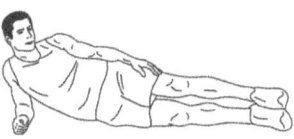

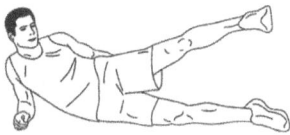

40 side leg raises

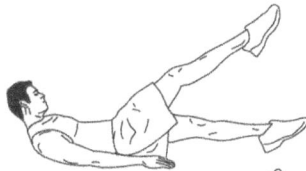

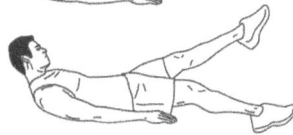

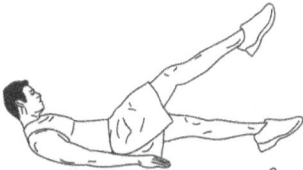

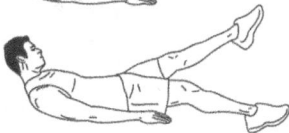

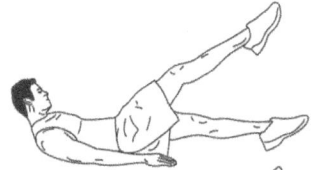

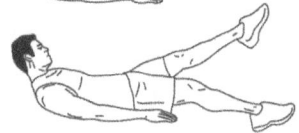

10 flutter kicks

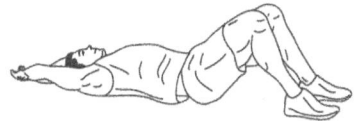

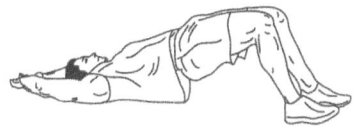

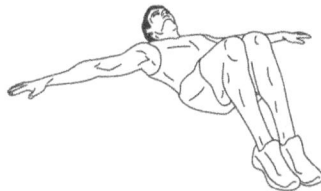

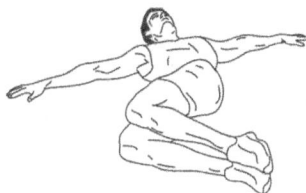

10 bridges

10 flutter kicks

10 knee rolls

10 flutter kicks

#57

Porter Workout

Focus: Cardiovascular system

Benefits: improved circulation, stronger lungs

PORTER

DAREBEE WORKOUT © darebee.com

LEVEL I 3 sets **LEVEL II** 5 sets **LEVEL III** 7 sets **REST** up to 2 minutes

20 march steps   **10** calf raises   **20** march steps

20 standing shoulder taps   **10** step jacks   **20** standing shoulder taps

#58

Posture Perfect Workout

Focus: Spine health

Benefits: stronger back & tendons

POSTURE PERFECT

DAREBEE WORKOUT © darebee.com

repeat 3 times | up to 2 minutes rest in between

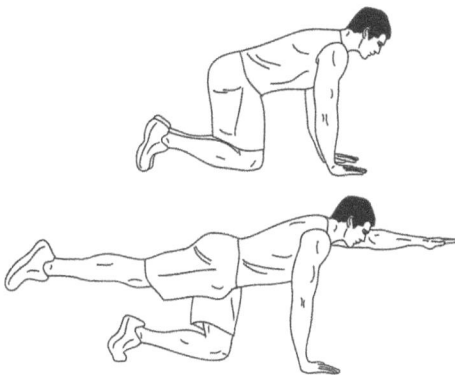

10 alt arm & leg raises

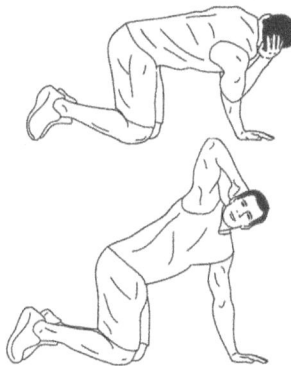

10 plank back rotations

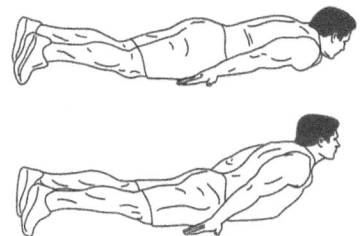

10 prone extensions

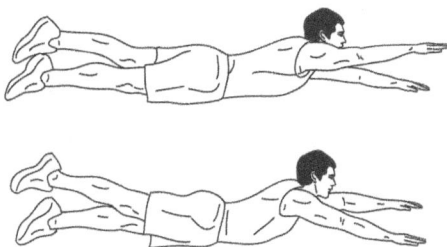

10 swimmers

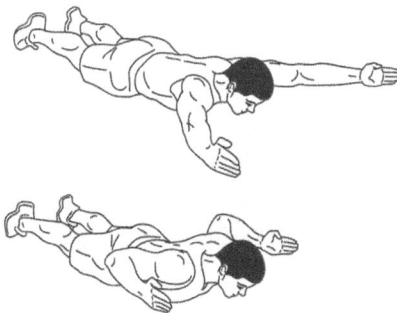

10 W-extensions

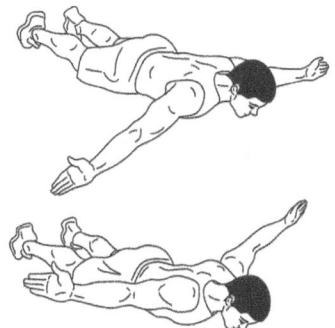

10 prone reverse fly

#59

Pressure Points Hand Workout

Focus: Hands & wrists

Benefits: improved hand dexterity

pressure
points

DAREBEE WORKOUT © darebee.com

Repeat each one for 10 seconds.

thenar press	palm rub	thumb root press
bottom index finger press	top little finger press	top thumb press

#60

Rainmaker Workout

Focus: Upper body

Benefits: improved range of motion, easier breathing

rainmaker

DAREBEE OFFICE WORKOUT © darebee.com

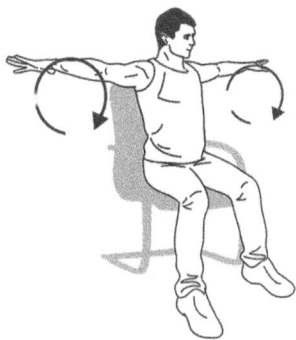

20 side circles

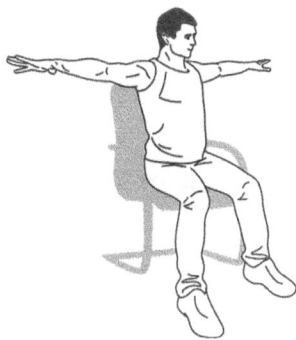

10-count hold

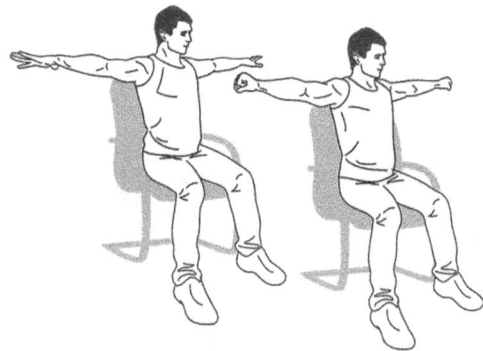

20 side clenches

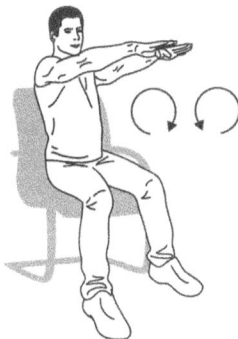

20 forward circles

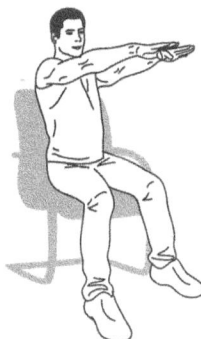

10-count hold

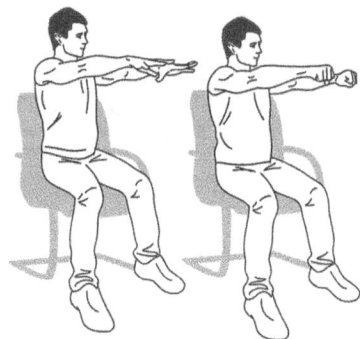

20 forward clenches

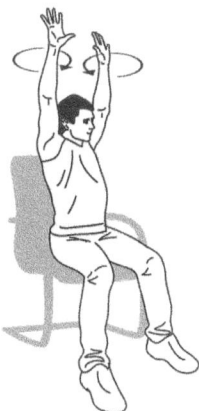

20 overhead circles

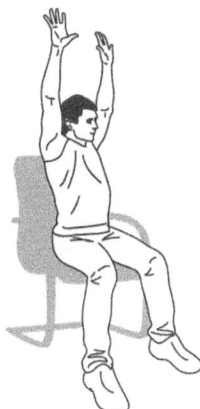

10-count hold

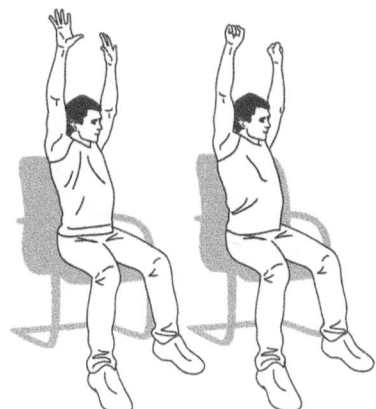

20 overhead clenches

#61

Real Workout

Focus: Balance & stability

Benefits: stronger tendons & lower body joints

KEEPING IT REAL

WORKOUT by DAREBEE © darebee.com

30 seconds rest between sets | No rest between exercises

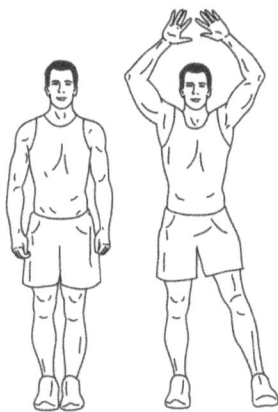

10 step jacks
x 3 sets in total

20 side leg raises
x 3 sets in total

20 back leg raises
x 3 sets in total

10 calf raises
x 3 sets in total

20 arm raises
x 3 sets in total

20 chest expansions
x 3 sets in total

#62

Recovery Workout

Focus: Agility

Benefits: improved posture, stronger spine & hips

RECOVERY WORKOUT

BY DAREBEE © darebee.com

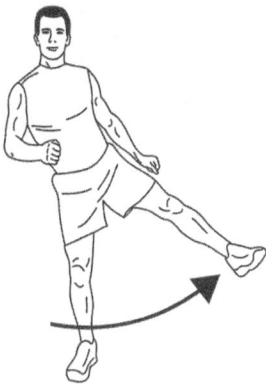

30 low side leg raises (right)

6 hip rotations (right)

30 low side leg raises (left)

6 hip rotations (left)

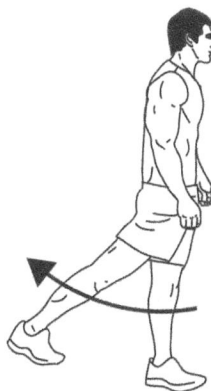

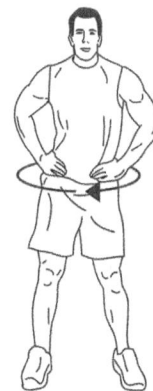

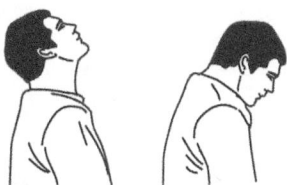

30 straight leg back swings (right leg)

6 hip rotations (right)

30 straight leg back swings (left leg)

6 hip rotations (left)

6 back and forth tilts   **6** side-to-side tilts   **6** neck rotations (3/3)

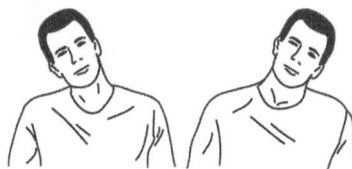

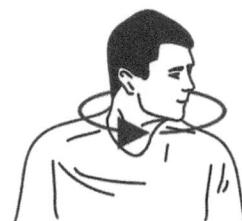

#63

Refresh Workout

Focus: Strength

Benefits: improved pecs, shoulders & calves

Refresh

DAREBEE WORKOUT © darebee.com

5 chest expansions

5 calf raises

10 chest expansions

10 calf raises

20 chest expansions

20 calf raises

done

#64

Regenerator Workout

Focus: Total body agility

Benefits: improved muscle tone, balance & posture

REGENERATOR

DAREBEE WORKOUT © darebee.com

LEVEL I 3 sets **LEVEL II** 5 sets **LEVEL III** 7 sets **REST** up to 2 minutes

10 step jacks

10 side leg raises

10 backward leg raises

10 alt chest expansions

10 chest expansions

10 arm circles

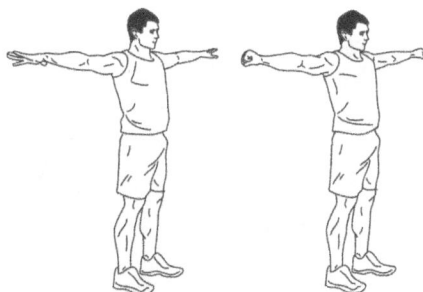

10 clench / unclench
arms to sides

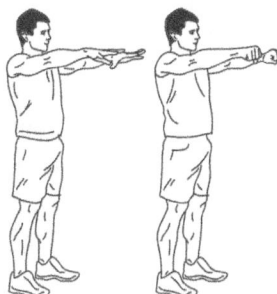

10 clench / unclench
arms forward

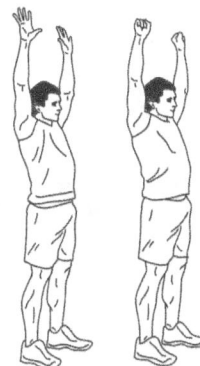

10 clench / unclench
arms overhead

#65

Regen Workout

Focus: cardiovascular system

Benefits: stronger legs, lungs and shoulders

RE-GEN

DAREBEE WORKOUT © darebee.com

LEVEL I 3 sets **LEVEL II** 5 sets **LEVEL III** 7 sets **REST** up to 2 minutes

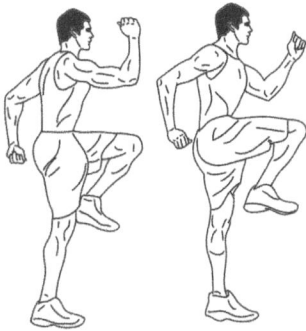

20 march steps

4 reverse lunges

20 march steps

20 raised arm circles

20 shoulder taps

20 raised arm circles

#66

Reset Stretch Workout

Focus: Flexibility

Benefits: improved muscle tone & range of motion

Reset Stretch

DAREBEE WORKOUT © **darebee.com**

20 seconds each exercise.

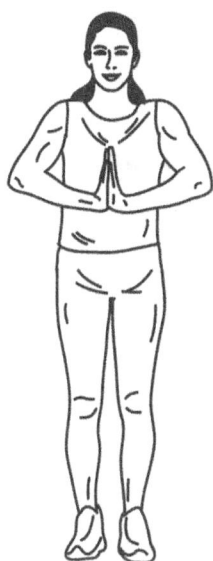

chest squeeze

tricep stretch

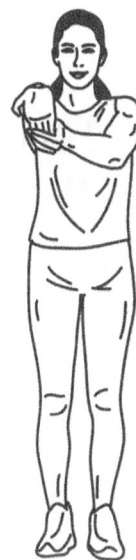

wrist stretch

back arch

tricep stretch (both arms)

overhead shoulder stretch

#67

Rest & Rec Workout

Focus: Spine & lower back

Benefits: greater flexibility & improved posture

REST & REC

DAREBEE
RECOVERY
WORKOUT
© darebee.com

20 knee-ins

10 back stretch #1

10 back stretch #2

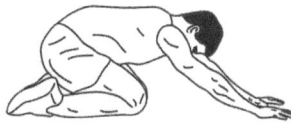

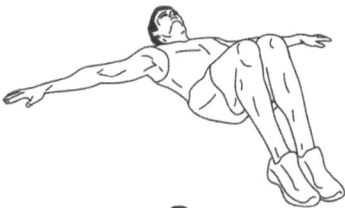

20 knee rolls

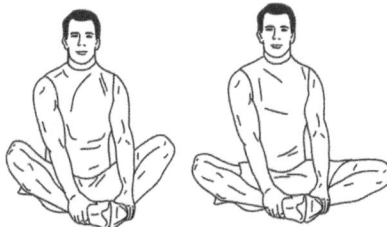

10 butterfly stretch

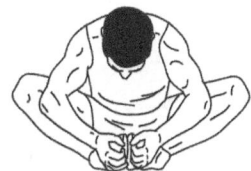

10 forward fold

#68

Rest & Repair Workout

Focus: Total body

Benefits: improves circulation, agility & posture

REST & REPAIR

DAREBEE WORKOUT © darebee.com

LEVEL I 3 sets **LEVEL II** 4 sets **LEVEL III** 5 sets **REST** up to 2 minutes

20 side leg raises

20 backward leg raises

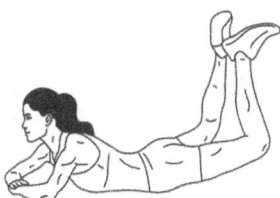

10 glute flex

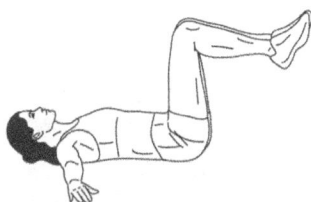

10 half wipers

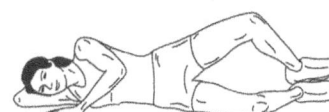

10 clamshells

#69

Right Side Bed Workout

Focus: Circulation & muscle preparedness

Benefits: Improved muscle tone & range of motion

the right side

DAREBEE 2-MINUTE BED WORKOUT © darebee.com

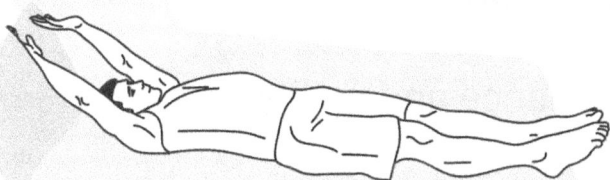

20sec "good morning" stretch

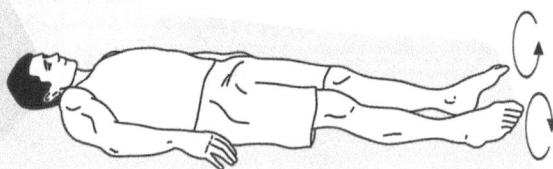

20sec in & out feet rotations

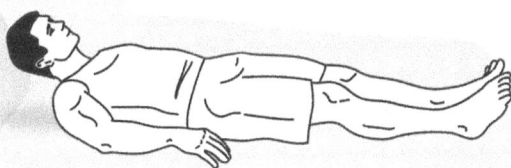

20sec slow head raises

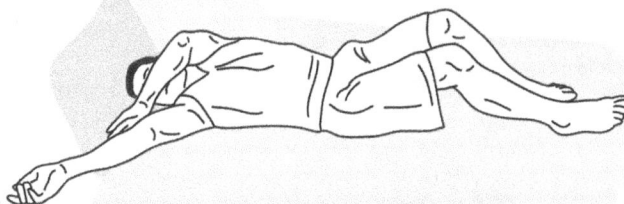

20sec slow side-to-side twists

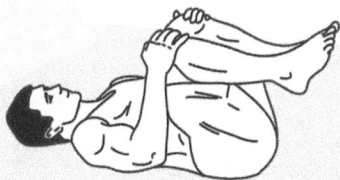

20sec knee-in pulse stretch

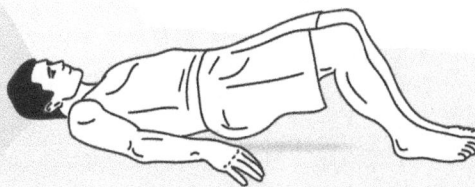

20sec bridge stretches

#70

Rookie Workout

Focus: Balance, strength, mobility

Benefits: Improved balance and agility

ROOKIE

DAREBEE WORKOUT © **darebee.com**

LEVEL I 3 sets **LEVEL II** 5 sets **LEVEL III** 7 sets **REST** up to 2 minutes

10 step jacks

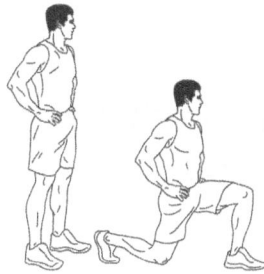

4 lunges

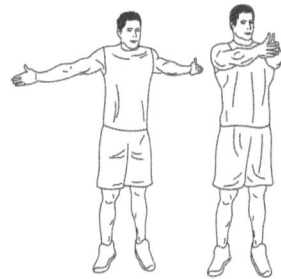

10 chest expansions

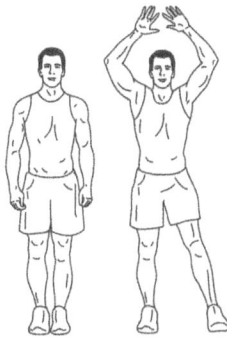

10 step jacks

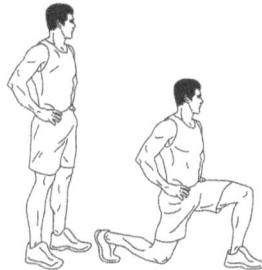

4 lunges

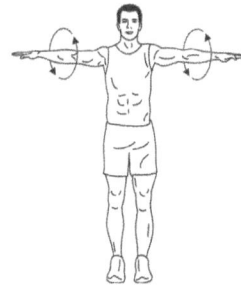

10 raised arm circles

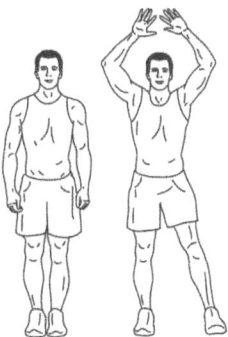

10 step jacks

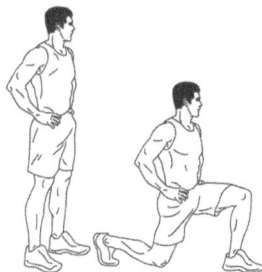

4 lunges

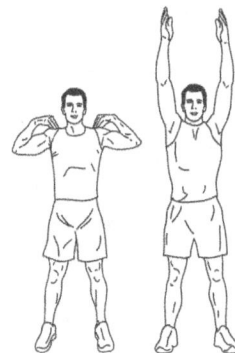

10 shoulder taps

#71

Rotator Cuff Workout

Focus: Shoulder mobility

Benefits: Upper body flexibility & strength

Rotator Cuff

DAREBEE REHAB WORKOUT © darebee.com
20 seconds each exercise.

arm twists

raised arms twists

half bow

full bow

elbow to torso

elbows in

#72

Roundabout Workout

Focus: Cardiovascular & aerobic health

Benefits: Improved circulation & endurance

Roundabout

DAREBEE WORKOUT © darebee.com

LEVEL I 3 sets **LEVEL II** 5 sets **LEVEL III** 7 sets **REST** up to 2 minutes

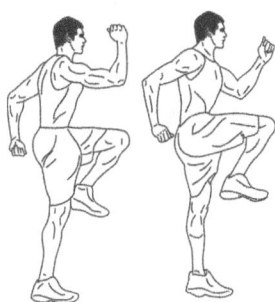

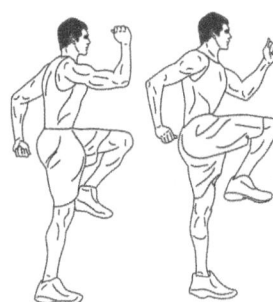

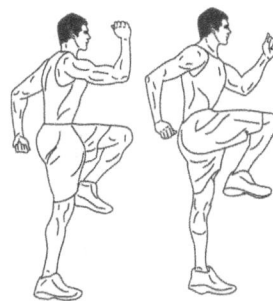

10 march steps

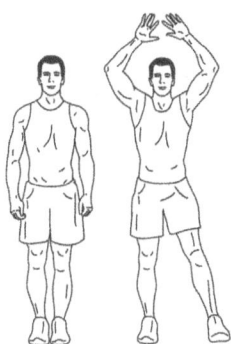

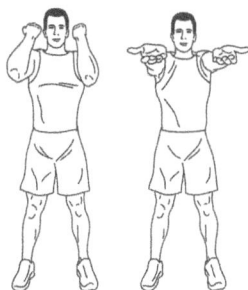

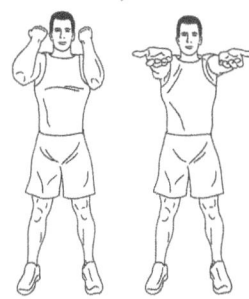

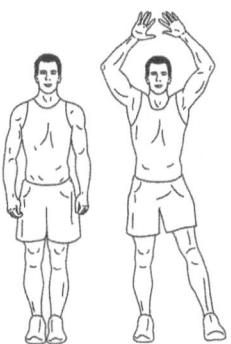

10 step jacks

10 march steps

10 bicep extensions

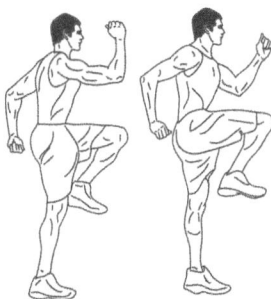

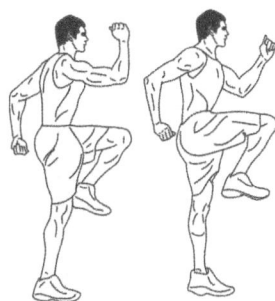

10 march steps

10 bicep extensions

10 march steps

10 step jacks

10 march steps

#73

Self Care Workout

Focus: Posture & flexibility

Benefits: Improved mobility & neck and spine health

self-care

DAREBEE WORKOUT © darebee.com

Hold each pose for 30 seconds then move on to the next one.
Repeat the sequence again on the other side.

1

2

3

4

5

6

7

8

9

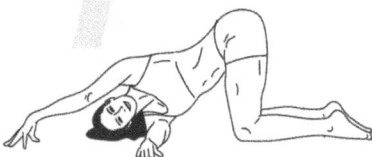

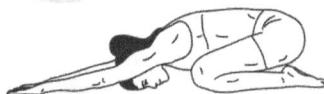

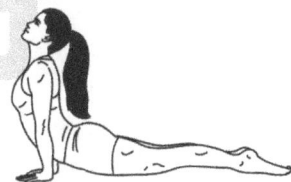

#74

Shoulder Stretch Workout

Focus: Upper body flexibility

Benefits: Improved upper body mobility & strength

shoulders
stretch

by DAREBEE © darebee.com
20 seconds each exercise.

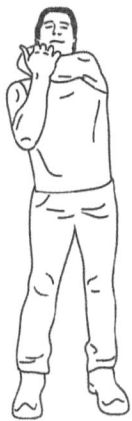

cross neck
stretch

shoulder
stretch

tricep
stretch

tricep
stretch #2

shoulders up
stretch

shoulder
& back stretch

behind back
lock stretch

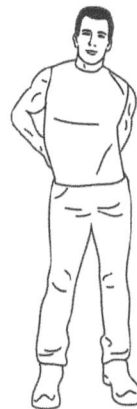

lock side pull
stretch

#75

Sitting Fix Workout

Focus: Range of motion

Benefits: Improved balance & flexibility

sitting fix

DAREBEE WORKOUT © darebee.com
20 seconds each exercise.

scapula stretch

shoulder stretch

corner chest stretch

quad stretch

hamstring stretch

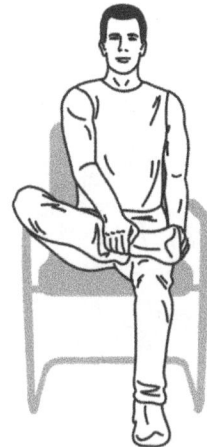

hip flexor stretch

#76

Slow Burn Workout

Focus: Tendon strength

Benefits: Improved balance, posture and stability

Slow Burn

DAREBEE WORKOUT © darebee.com

repeat 3 times with 2 minutes rest in between

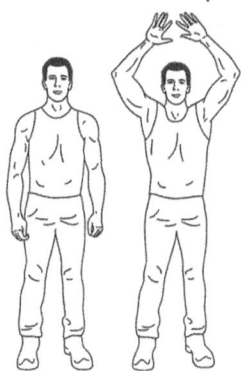

10 arm raises

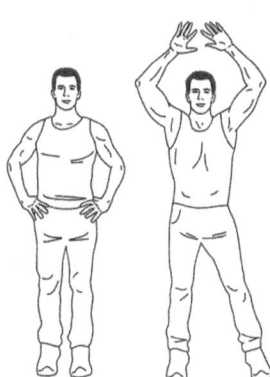

10 step jacks

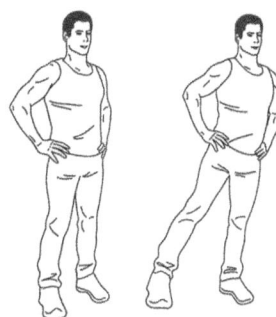

20 side leg raises

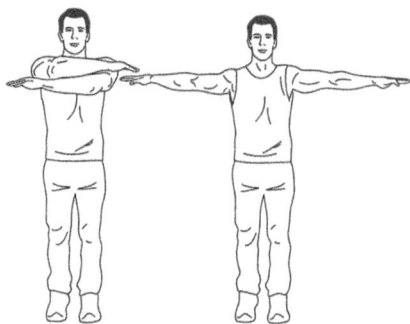

10 chest extensions

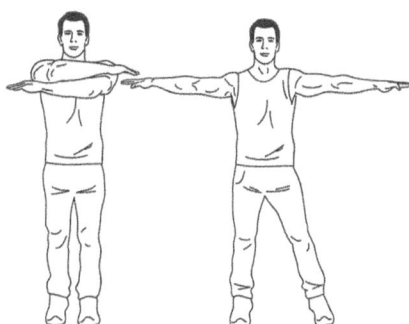

10 step chest extensions

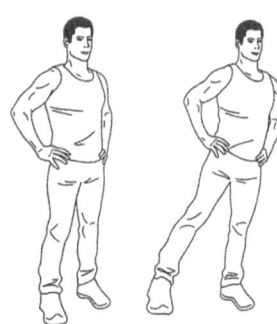

20 side leg raises

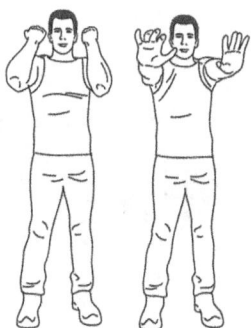

10 bicep extensions

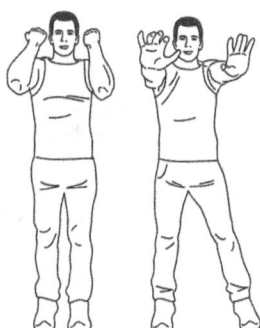

10 step bicep extensions

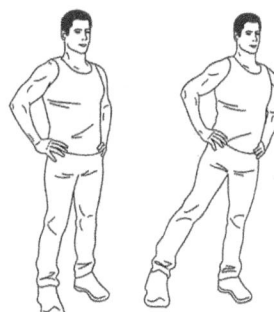

20 side leg raises

#77

Something I Can Do Workout

Focus: Cardiovascular & aerobic systems

Benefits: Improved mobility, posture & endurance

SOMETHING I CAN *actually* DO

DAREBEE WORKOUT © darebee.com

LEVEL I 3 sets **LEVEL II** 5 sets **LEVEL III** 7 sets **REST** up to 2 minutes

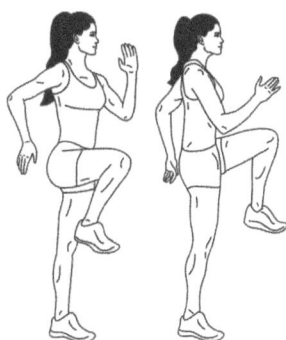

20 march steps

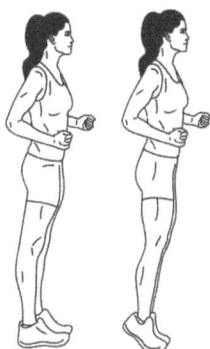

5 calf raises

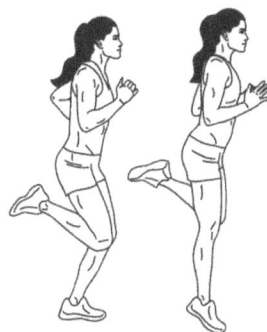

20 butt kicks

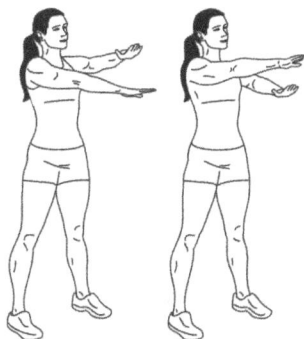

20 arm scissors

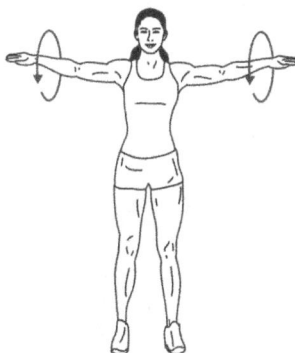

10 raised arm circles

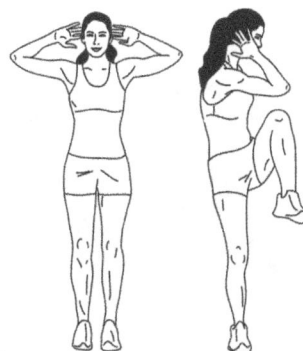

10 knee-to-elbows

#78

Sore Feet Workout

Focus: Well-being

Benefits: Improved circulation & better feet health

sore feet

DAREBEE WORKOUT © darebee.com
20 seconds each exercise.

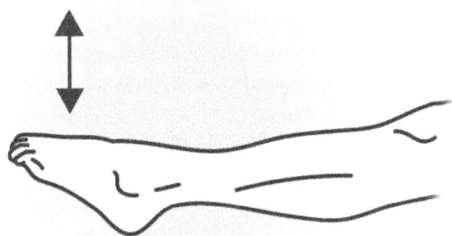

up and down tilts

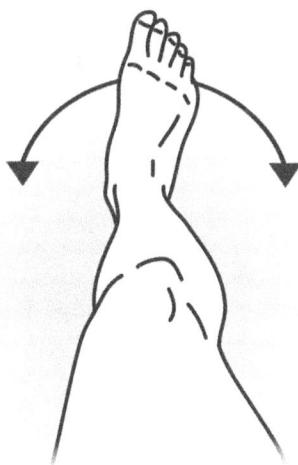

side-to-side tilts

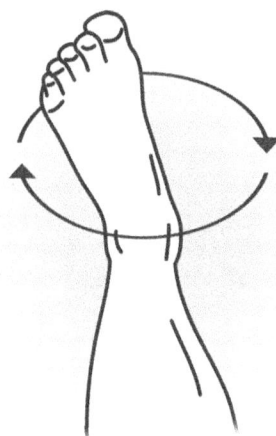

rotations

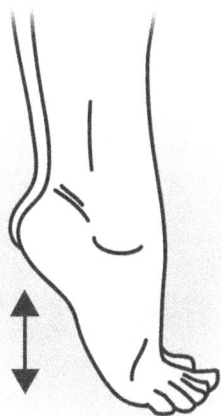

calf raises

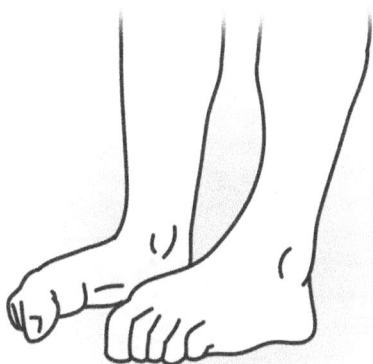

toe curls

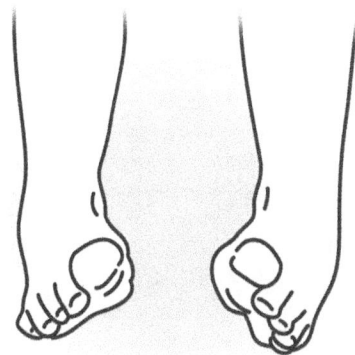

side tilts

#79

Sore Neck Workout

Focus: Neck flexibility

Benefits: Improved range of motion & better neck strength

sore neck

DAREBEE WORKOUT © darebee.com
20 seconds each exercise.

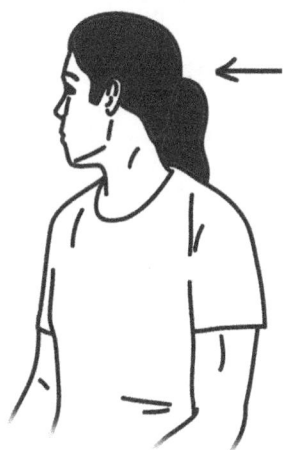

side-to-side turns

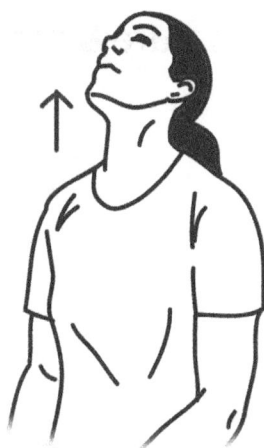

up & down nods

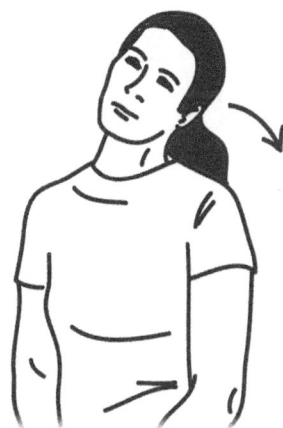

side-to-side tilts

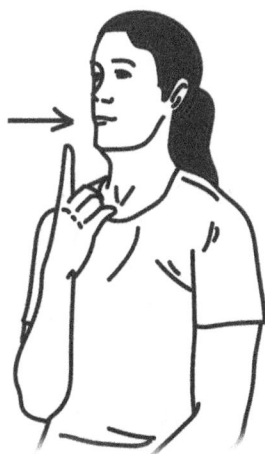

head back

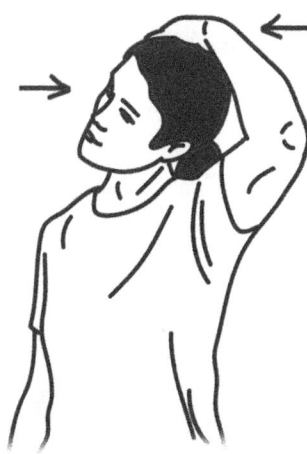

side stretch
(resistance)

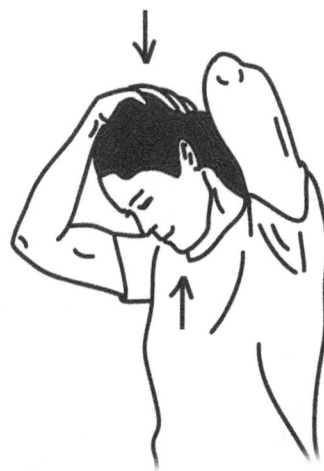

forward stretch
(resistance)

#80

Spine Mobility Workout

Focus: Spine flexibility

Benefits: Improved posture & resistance to fatigue

spine
mobility

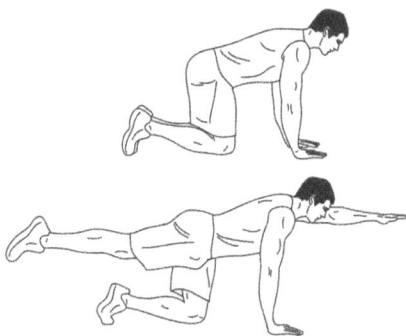

10 alt arm/ leg extensions
3 sets in total
30 sec rest in between

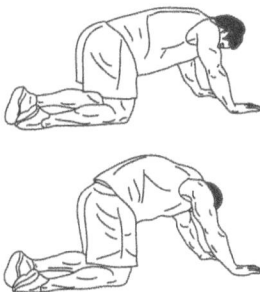

10 back arches
3 sets in total
30 sec rest in between

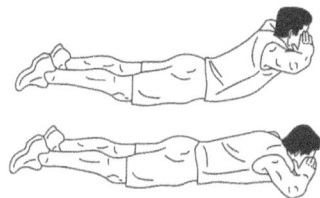

10 back extensions
3 sets in total
30 sec rest in between

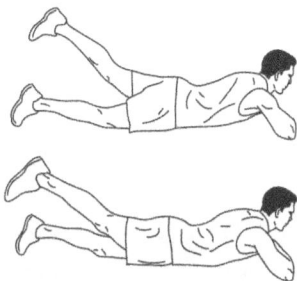

10 reverse flutter kicks
3 sets in total
30 sec rest in between

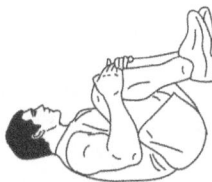

10-count knee hug stretch
3 sets in total
30 sec rest in between

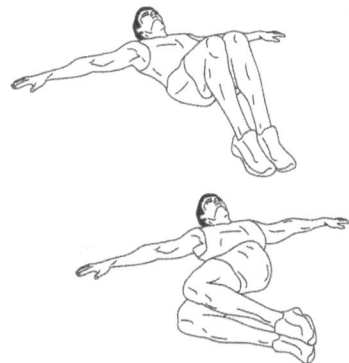

10 knee rolls
3 sets in total
30 sec rest in between

#81

Stapler Workout

Focus: Hand & forearm strength

Benefits: Improved grip strength & overall health

STAPLER

DAREBEE WORKOUT © darebee.com

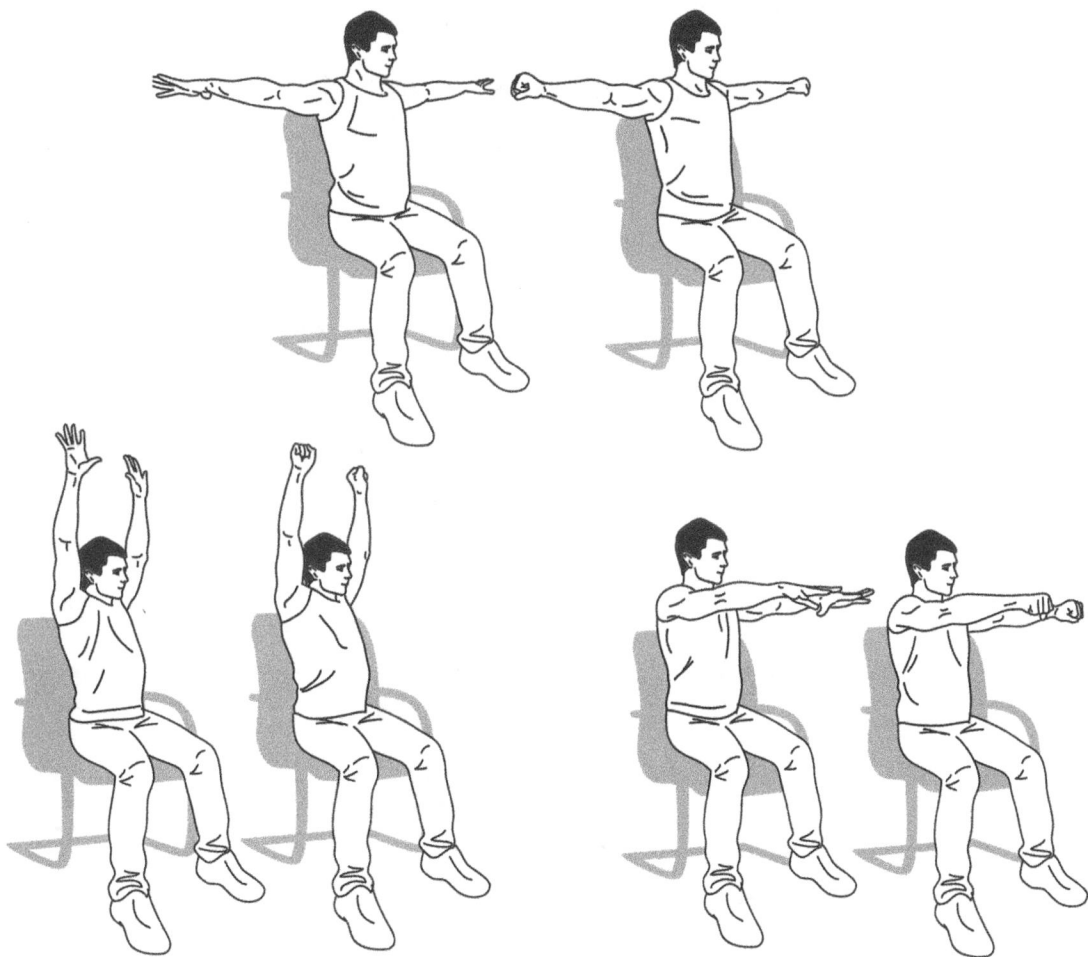

20 arms to the side clench / unclench

20 arms overhead clench / unclench

20 arms to the front clench / unclench

#82

Starting Point Workout

Focus: Balance & agility

Benefits: Improved posture, agility & core stability

STARTING
POINT

DAREBEE WORKOUT © darebee.com

LEVEL I 3 sets **LEVEL II** 5 sets **LEVEL III** 7 sets **REST** up to 2 minutes

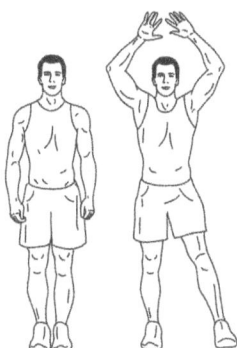

10 step jacks

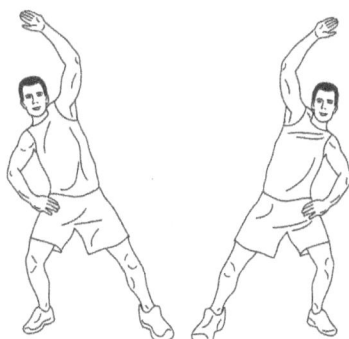

10 side jacks

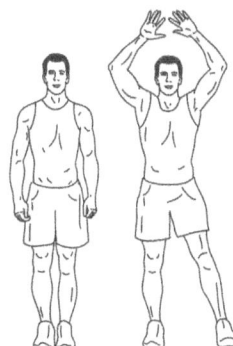

10 step jacks

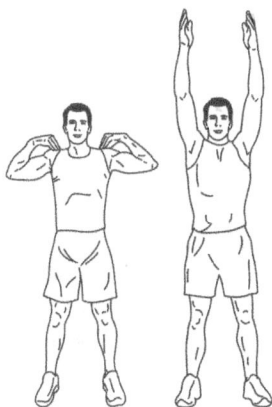

10 shoulder taps

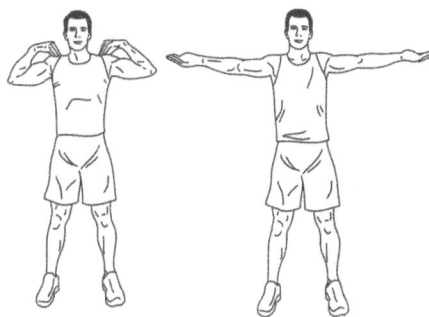

10 side shoulder taps

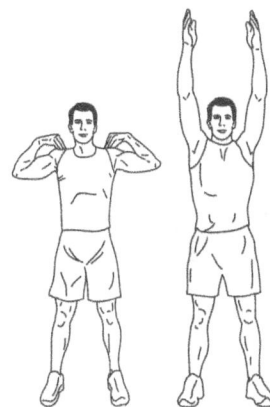

10 shoulder taps

#83

Steamroller Workout

Focus: Lower body strength and agility

Benefits: Improved lower body strength & coordination

STEAMROLLER

DAREBEE WORKOUT © darebee.com

LEVEL I 3 sets **LEVEL II** 5 sets **LEVEL III** 7 sets **REST** up to 2 minutes

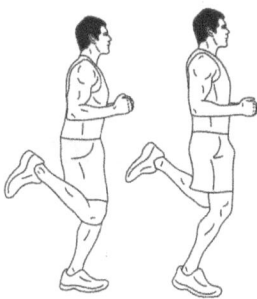

10 butt kicks

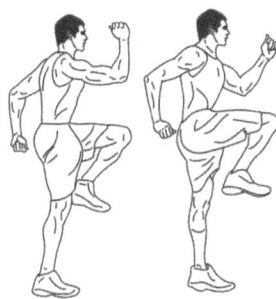

10 march steps

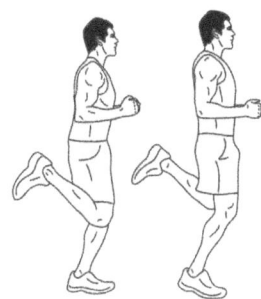

10 butt kicks

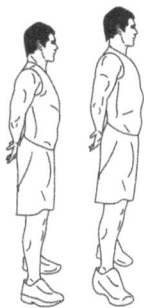

5 calf raises

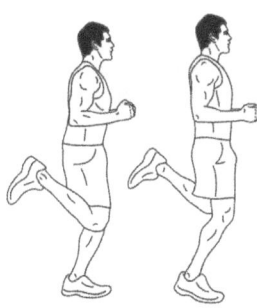

10 butt kicks

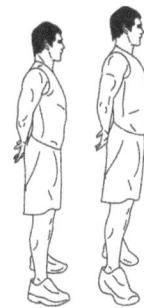

5 calf raises

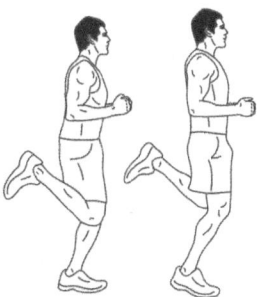

10 butt kicks

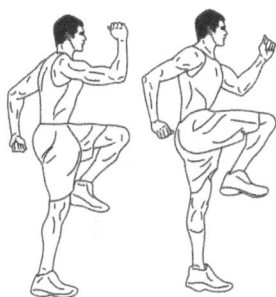

10 march steps

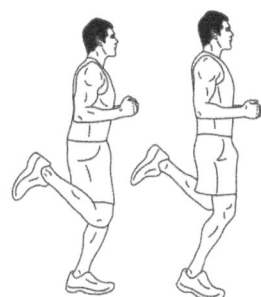

10 butt kicks

#84

Stiff Neck Workout

Focus: Neck suppleness

Benefits: Relaxed neck muscles & improved circulation

stiff neck

DAREBEE WORKOUT © darebee.com
20 seconds each exercise.

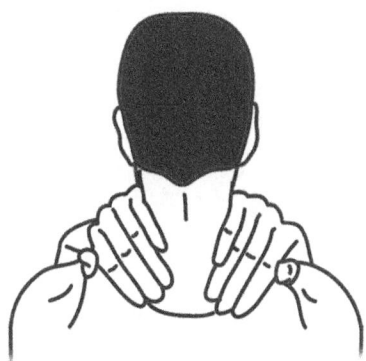

neck massage

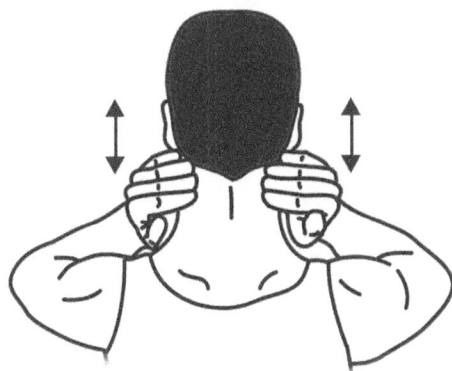

up and down rows

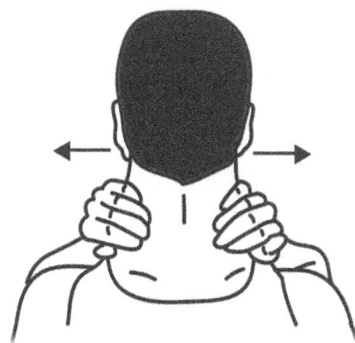

opposite rows

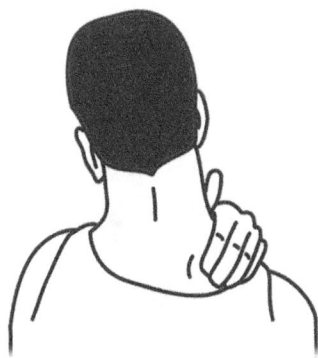

shoulder massage

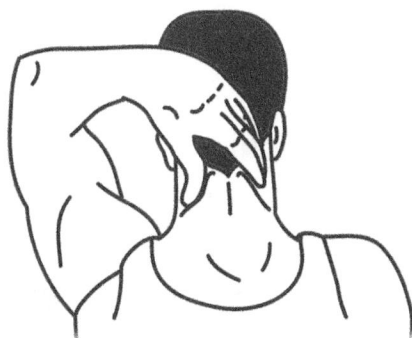

grip slides

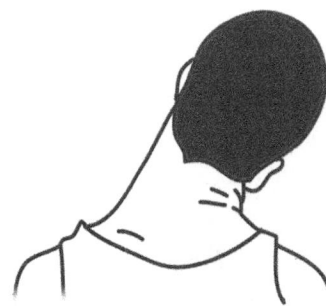

side-to-side tilts

#85

Stronger Arms Workout

Focus: Chest & shoulders strength

Benefits: Increased upper body strength

stronger arms

DAREBEE WORKOUT © darebee.com

LEVEL I 3 sets **LEVEL II** 5 sets **LEVEL III** 7 sets **REST** up to 2 minutes

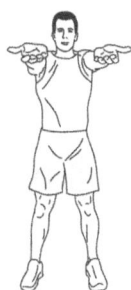

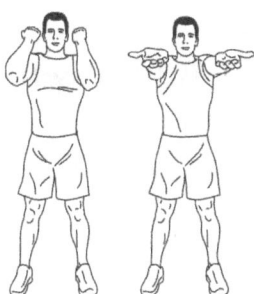

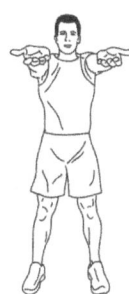

10-count hold   **20** bicep extensions   **10-count** hold

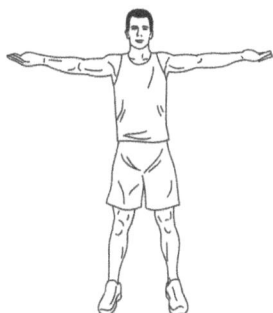

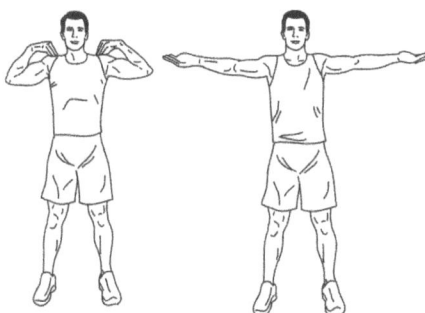

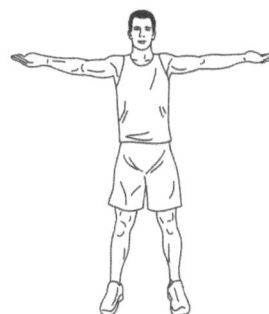

10-count hold   **20** side shoulder taps   **10-count** hold

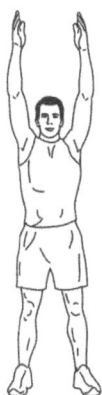

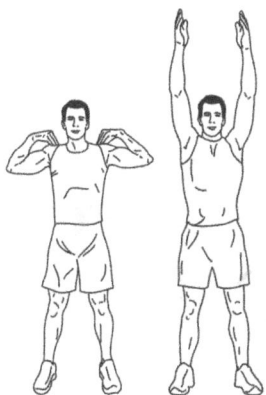

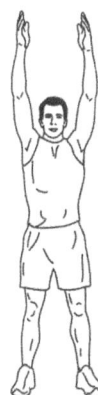

10-count hold   **20** shoulder taps   **10-count** hold

#86

Sun Salutation Chair Workout

Focus: Agility & mobility

Benefits: Improved circulation & overall flexibility

Sun Salutation
chair edition

DAREBEE WORKOUT © darebee.com

Hold each pose for 10 seconds and move to the next one.

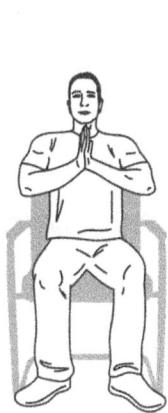

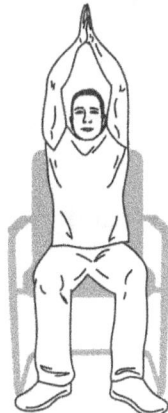

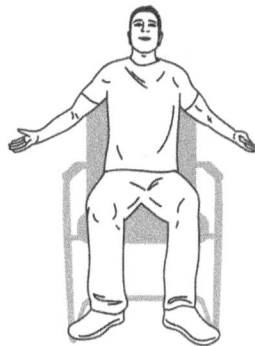

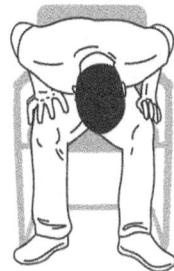

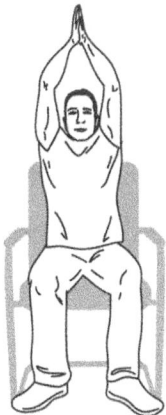

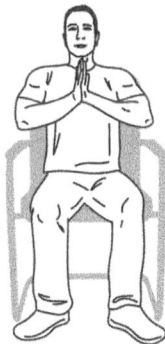

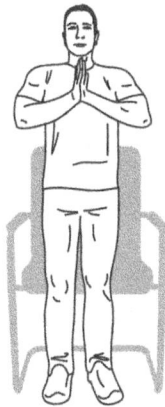

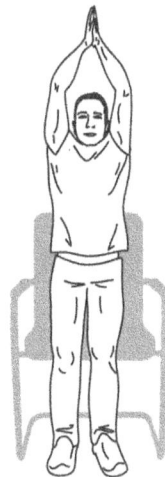

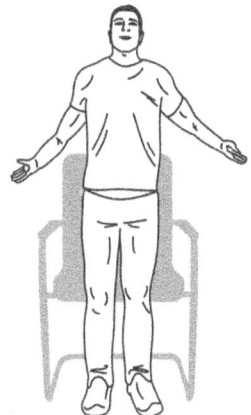

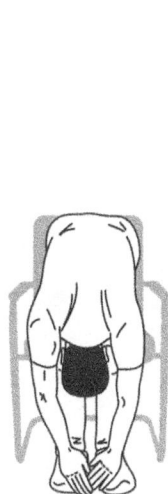

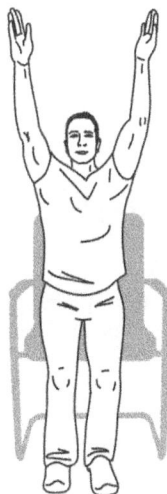

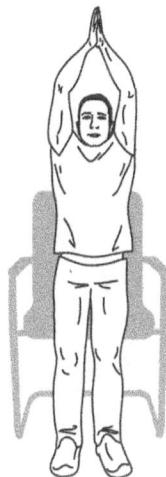

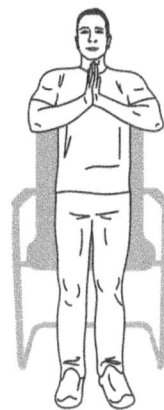

#87

Super Easy Workout

Focus: Agility and flexibility

Benefits: Improved mobility and upper body range of motion

SUPER EASY

DAREBEE WORKOUT © darebee.com

LEVEL I 3 sets **LEVEL II** 5 sets **LEVEL III** 7 sets **REST** up to 2 minutes

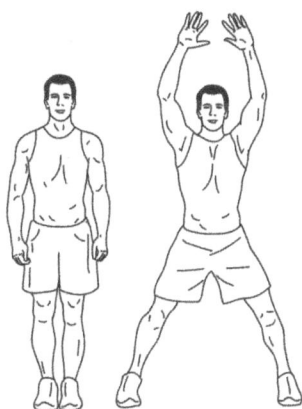

10 jumping jacks

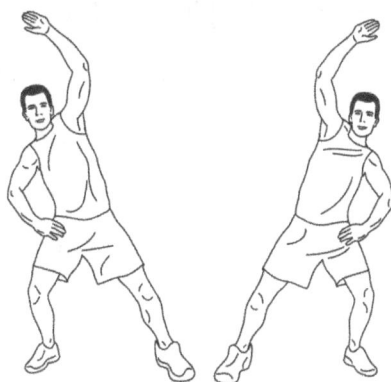

10 side jacks

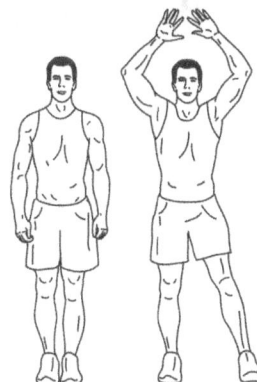

10 step jacks

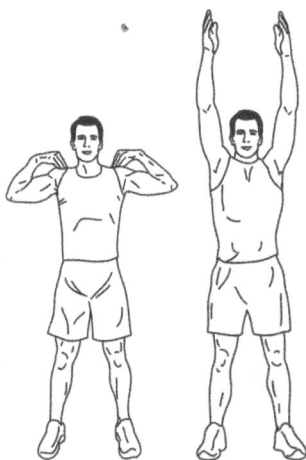

10 shoulder taps

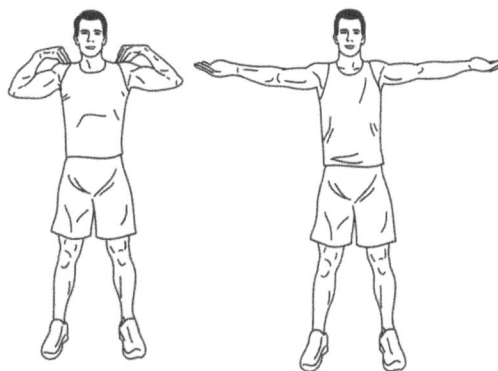

10 side shoulder taps

#88

Tai Chi Workout

Focus: Cardiovascular system

Benefits: Improved agility, joint strength and coordination

Tai Chi

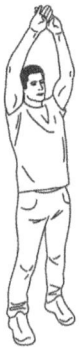

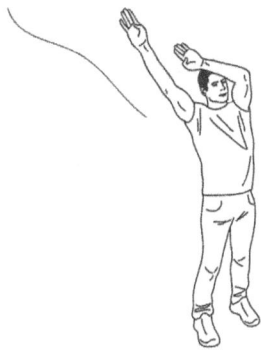

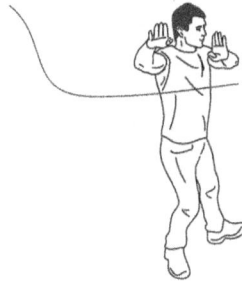

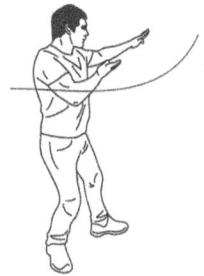

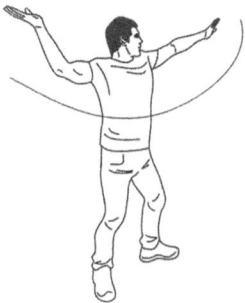

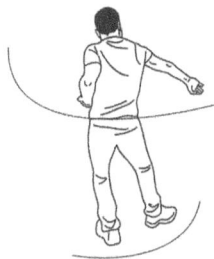

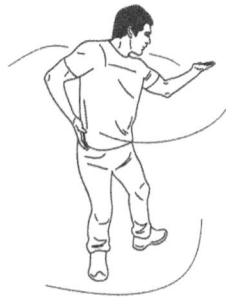

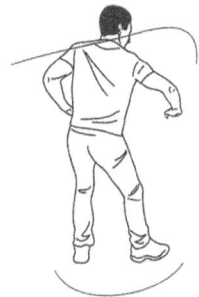

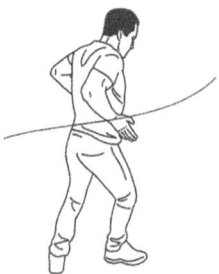

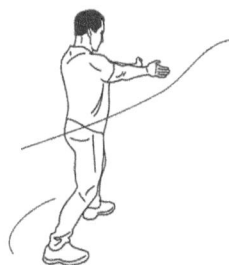

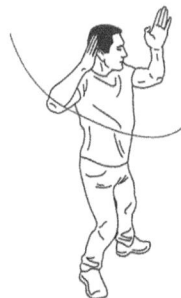

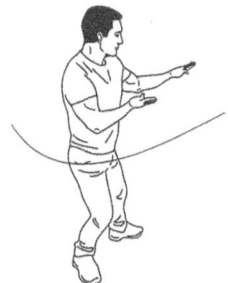

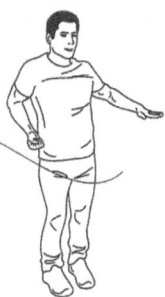

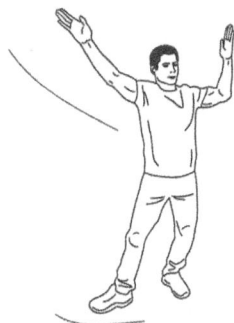

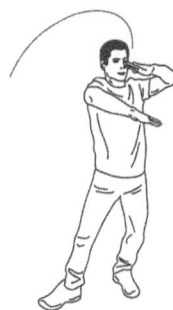

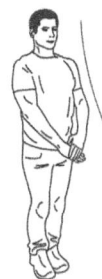

#89

Toy Soldier Workout

Focus: Aerobic system

Benefits: Improved endurance and body fat reduction

TOY SOLDIER

DAREBEE WORKOUT © darebee.com

LEVEL I 3 sets **LEVEL II** 5 sets **LEVEL III** 7 sets **REST** up to 2 minutes

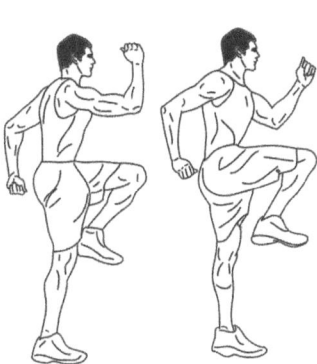

30sec march steps

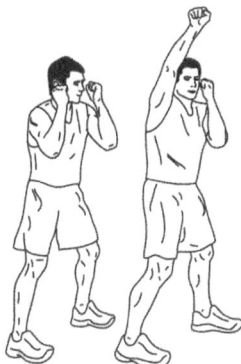

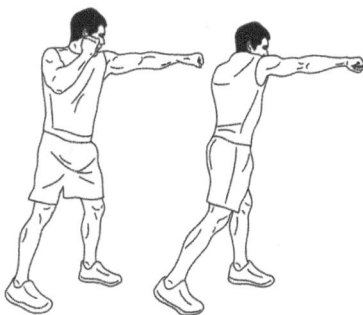

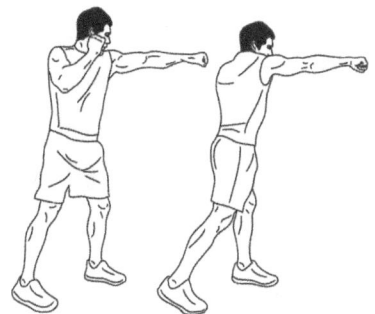

30sec overhead punches

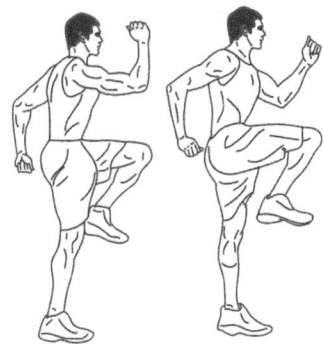

30sec march steps

30sec punches

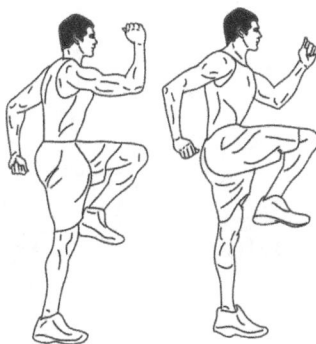

30sec march steps

30sec punches

#90

Unwind Workout

Focus: Flexibility

Benefits: Improved spine and joint health

UNWIND

DAREBEE WORKOUT © darebee.com

#1 Slowly shift from *Cat Pose to Cow Pose* continuously for 30 seconds.
#2 Breathe out quickly 5 times then hold the pose.
Hold each pose after #2 for 30 seconds.

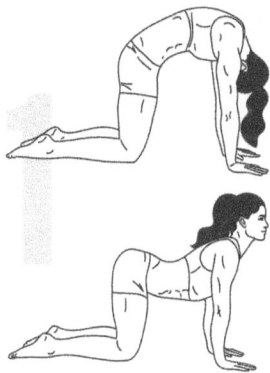

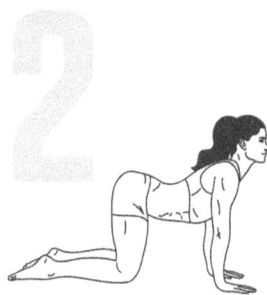

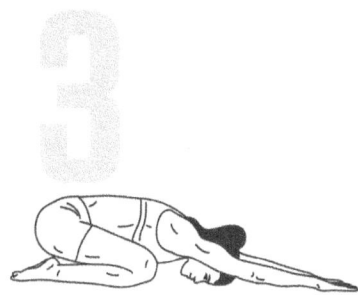

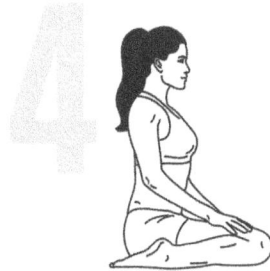

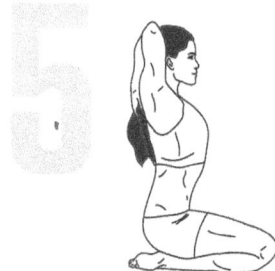

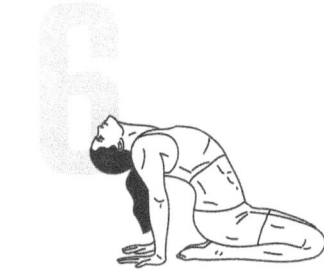

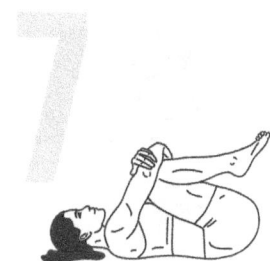

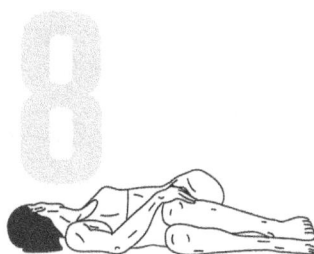

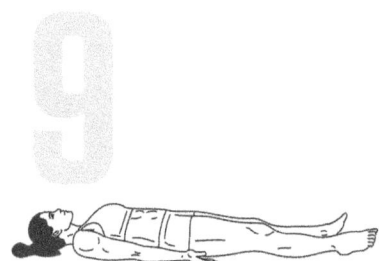

#91

Upperbody Mobility Workout

Focus: Upper body flexibility
Benefits: Improved range of movement

upperbody
mobility

DAREBEE WORKOUT
© darebee.com
repeat 3 times
1 minute rest

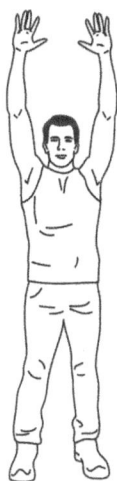

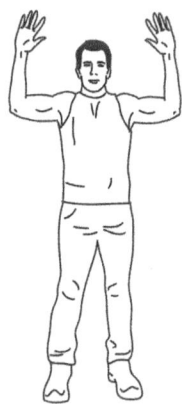

20 W-extensions

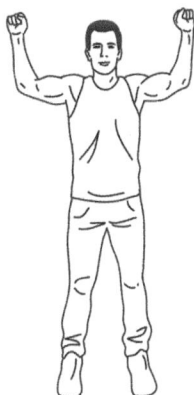

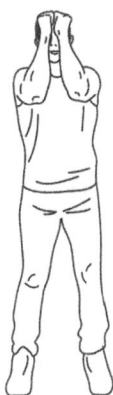

20 elbow clicks

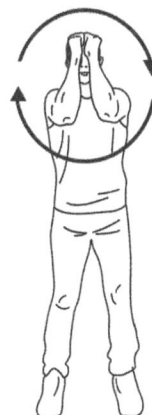

20 elbows together rotations

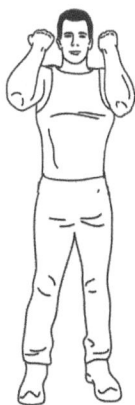

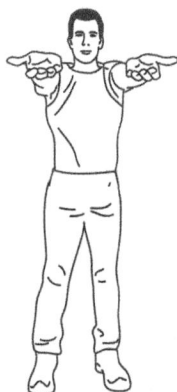

20 bicep extensions

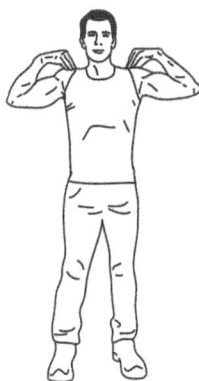

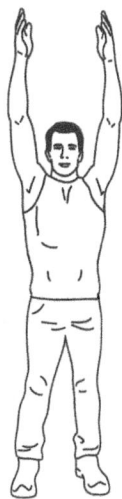

20 shoulder taps

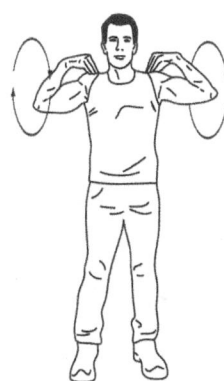

20 elbow rotations

#92

Upperbody Stretch Workout

Focus: Flexibility

Benefits: Improved mobility and range of movement

upperbody
stretch

by DAREBEE © darebee.com
20 seconds each exercise.

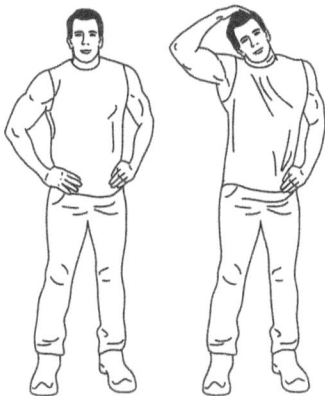

neck stretches

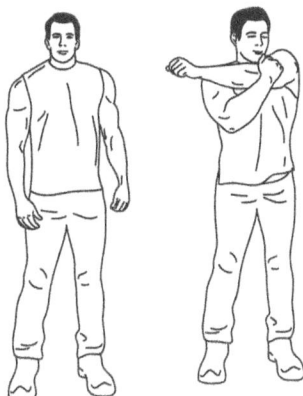

shoulder stretches

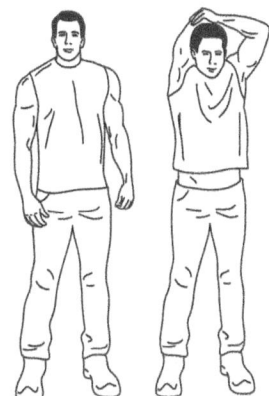

tricep stretches

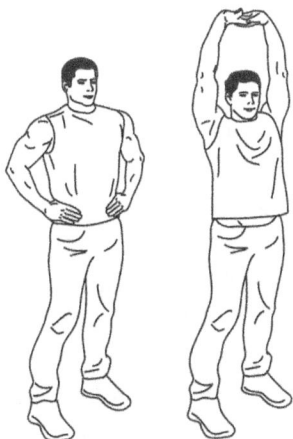

back & shoulders stretches

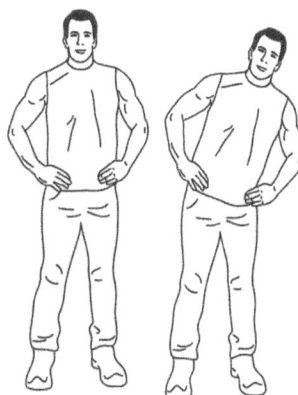

side bends

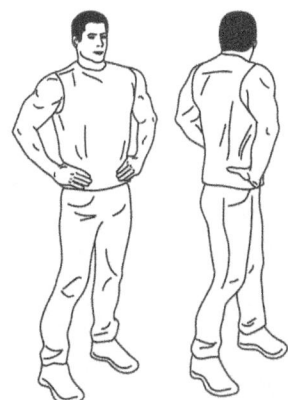

torso rotations

#93

Upperbody Works Workout

Focus: Upper body agility

Benefits: Improved tendon strength and muscle tone

upperbody
works

DAREBEE WORKOUT © darebee.com

LEVEL I 3 sets **LEVEL II** 4 sets **LEVEL III** 5 sets **REST** up to 2 minutes

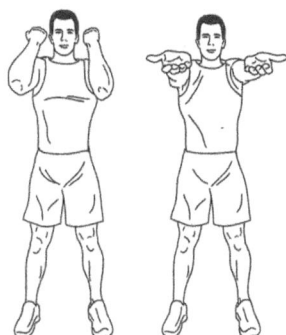

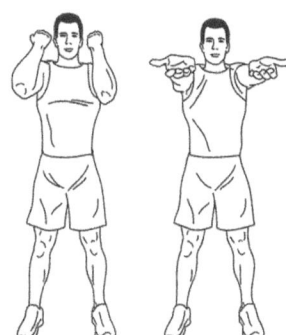

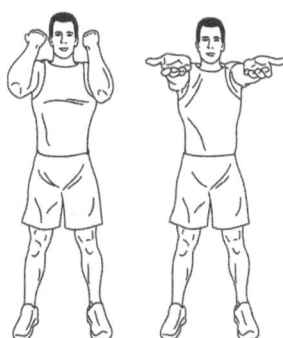

20 bicep extensions   **20** standing shoulder taps   **20** bicep extensions

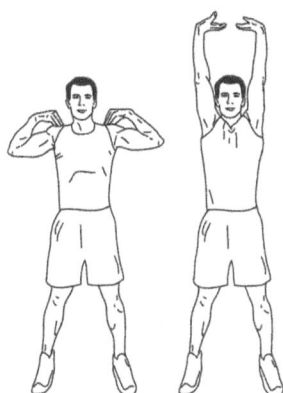

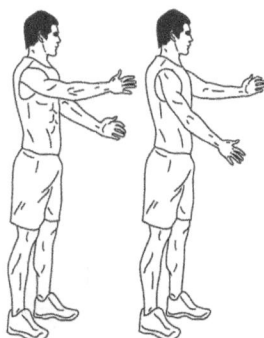

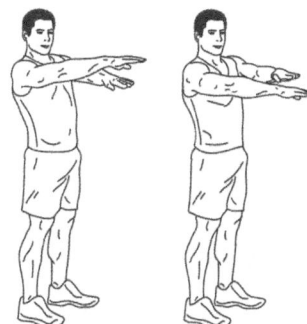

20 scissors chops   **20** bicep extensions   **20** arm scissors

#94

Vortex Workout

Focus: Upper body

Benefits: Improved muscle tone and shoulder strength

vortex

DAREBEE WORKOUT © darebee.com

LEVEL I 3 sets **LEVEL II** 4 sets **LEVEL III** 5 sets **REST** up to 2 minutes

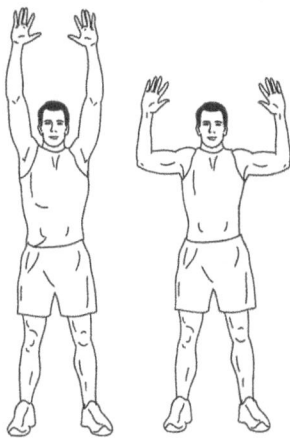

20 standing W-extensions

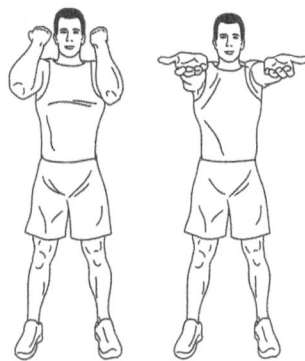

20 bicep extensions

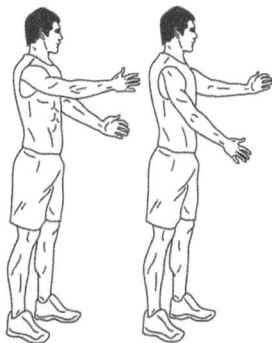

20 scissor chops

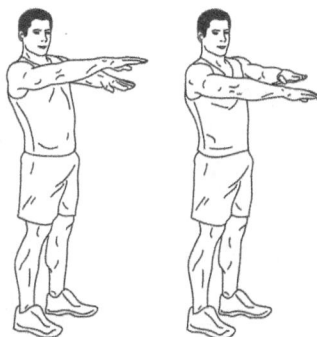

20 arm scissors

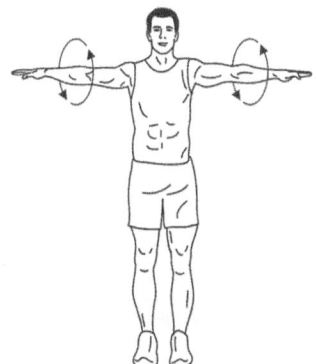

20 raised arm circles

#95

Walker Workout

Focus: Cardiovascular system

Benefits: Improved posture and lower body strength and stability

walker

WORKOUT by DAREBEE © darebee.com
Repeat 3 times in total | 2 minutes rest between sets

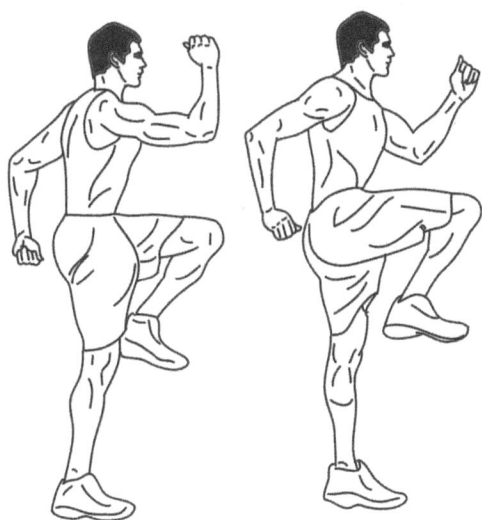

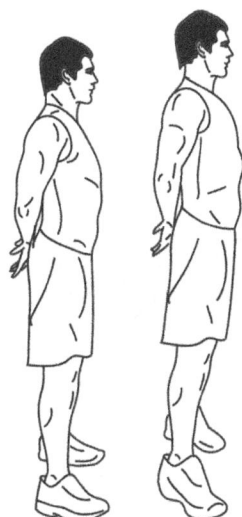

20 march steps

5 calf raises

20 march steps

5 calf raises

20 march steps

5 calf raises

20 march steps

5 calf raises

20 march steps

5 calf raises

#96

Walk It Off Workout

Focus: Cardiovascular system

Benefits: Improved blood flow circulation, increased agility

WALK IT OFF

DAREBEE WORKOUT © darebee.com

LEVEL I 3 sets **LEVEL II** 5 sets **LEVEL III** 7 sets **REST** up to 2 minutes

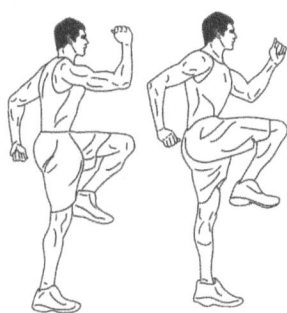

10 march steps

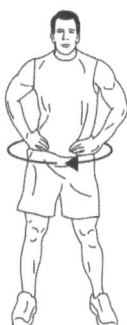

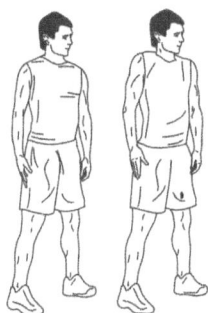

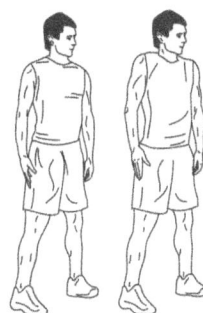

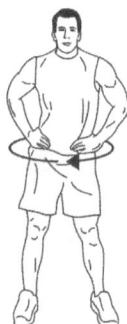

10 hip rotations

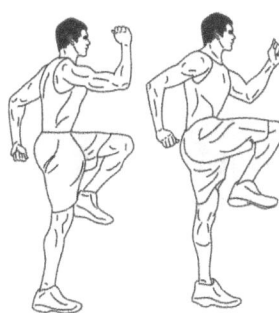

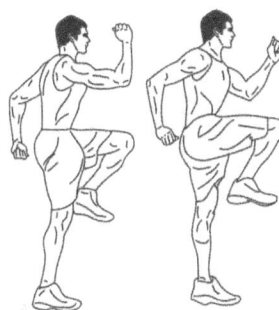

10 march steps

10 shoulder shrugs

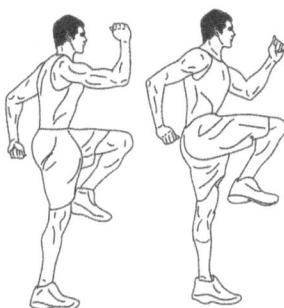

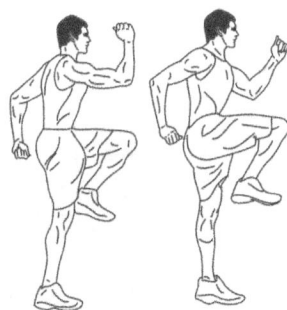

10 march steps

10 shoulder shrugs

10 march steps

10 hip rotations

10 march steps

#97

Wizard Workout

Focus: Upper body

Benefits: Improved shoulder strength and upper body mobility

WIZARD

DAREBEE WORKOUT © darebee.com

LEVEL I 3 sets **LEVEL II** 4 sets **LEVEL III** 5 sets

REST up to 2 minutes

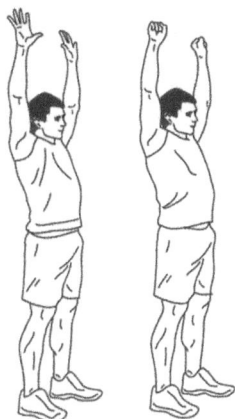

20 clench/unclench overhead

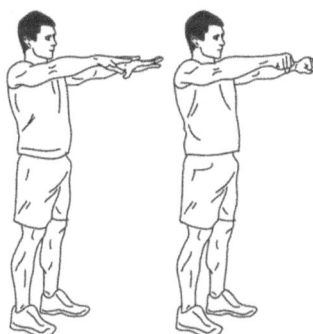

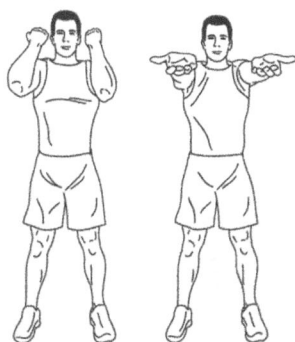

20 clench/unclench

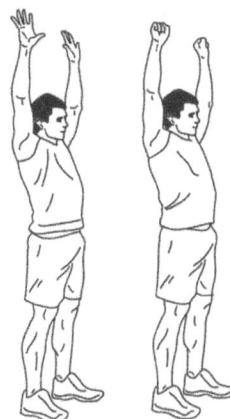

20 clench/unclench overhead

20 bicep extensions

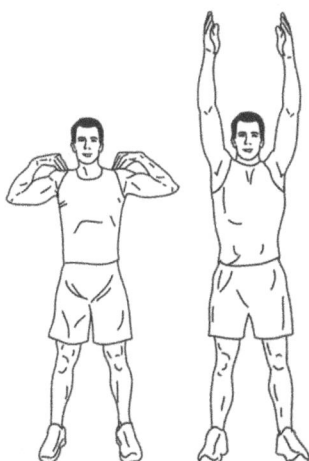

20 standing shoulder taps

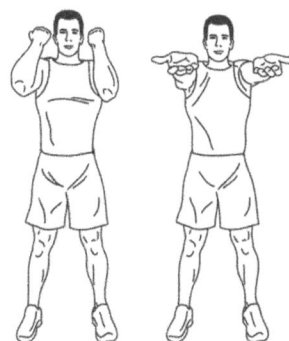

20 bicep extensions

#98

Wrist Pain Workout

Focus: Wrists

Benefits: Improved tendon strength and wrist mobility

wrist pain

DAREBEE WORKOUT © darebee.com
20 seconds each exercise.
Repeat every couple of hours.

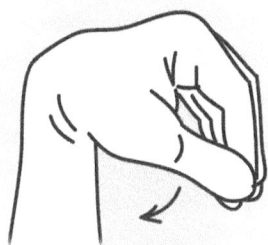

wrist curl

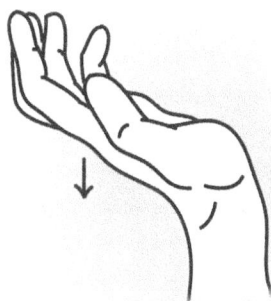

tilt back

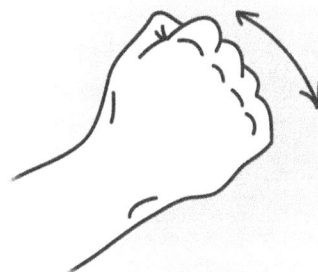

"hammer"

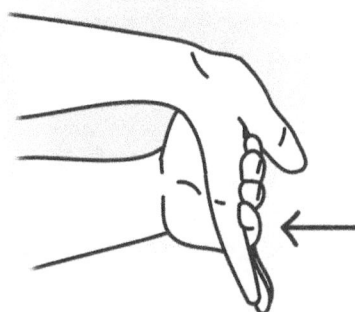

wrist stretch

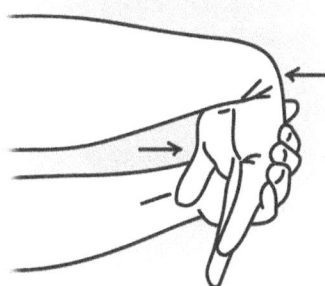

resistance press

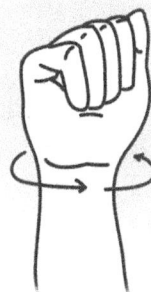

fist rotations

#99

Yoga Flow Workout

Focus: Flexibility

Benefits: Improved cardiovascular health and posture

yoga
flow

DAREBEE WORKOUT
© darebee.com
Hold each pose
for 20 seconds.

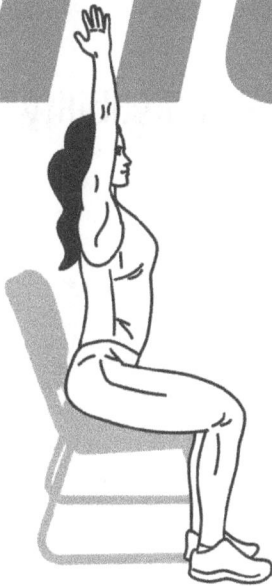

reach

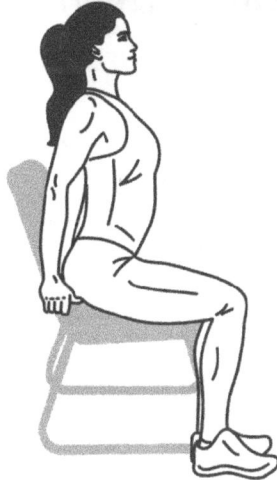

shoulders back

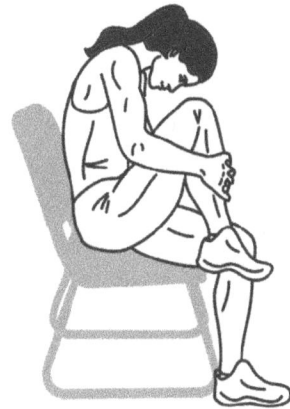

knee bend to cobra

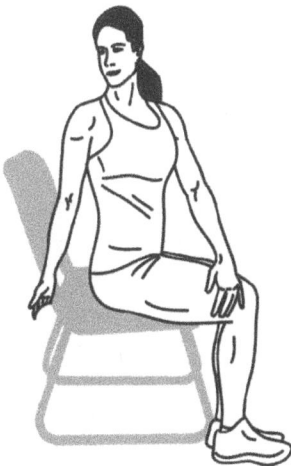

twist

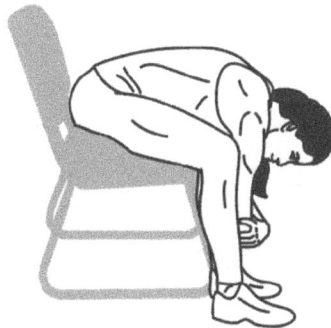

forward bend

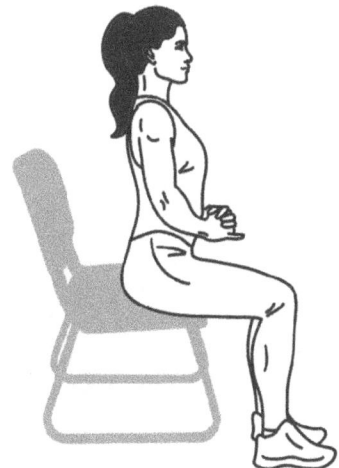

straight back

#100

Zen Workout

Focus: Inner peace

Benefits: Improved breathing, concentration and flexibility

ZEN

Hold each pose for 30 seconds then move on to the next one.

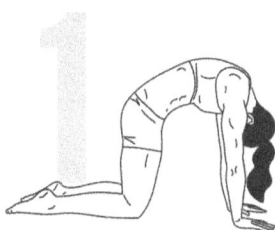

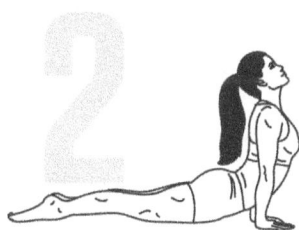

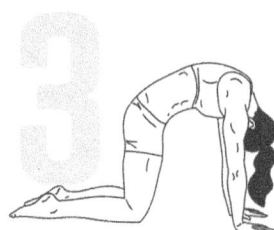

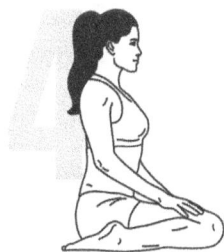

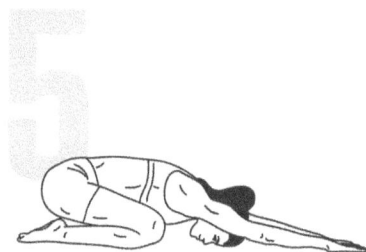

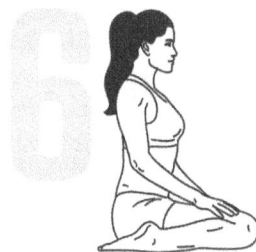

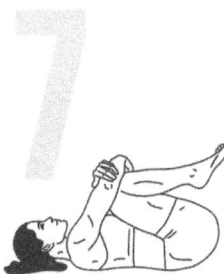

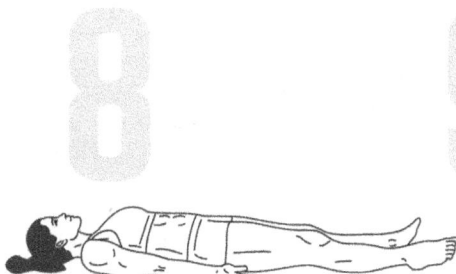

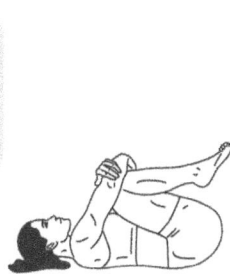

1

2

3

4

5

6

7

8

9

www.ingramcontent.com/pod-product-compliance
Lightning Source LLC
Chambersburg PA
CBHW080848270326

41935CB00012B/1551